AGING REVERSED

How We Age and How to Stay Younger Longer (The Science of Aging)

Wendy Owen - Dip.HHT (HHC)

Aging Reversed - Wendy Owen

Third Edition – Revised December 2020

The number one question I've been asked recently is, "How can I lose some weight? I've tried everything, and nothing is working!"

There are three main reasons why this could be happening. I've put them in a short and

informative guide – just type in the link below:

https://www.naturalhealthpublishing.org/balance-blood-sugar/

Copyright

21 Callistemon Court, Greenbank, Queensland, Australia, 4124

https://www.NaturalHealthPublishing.org

© 2020 Wendy Owen

Health Disclaimer

All material on this website is provided for your information only and may not be construed as medical advice or instruction. No action or inaction should be taken based solely on the contents of this information; instead, readers should consult appropriate health professionals on any matter relating to their health and well-being.

The information and opinions expressed here are believed to be accurate, based on the best judgement available to the author, and readers who fail to consult with appropriate health authorities assume the risk of any injuries.

Contents

Chapter 1 - My Story

"At age 20, we worry about what others think of us. At age 40, we don't care what they think of us. At age 60, we discover they haven't been thinking of us at all." - Ann Landers

We are not controlled by our age. Yes, we will grow older, but we have a lot of control over how old we feel.

Getting older shouldn't be something we dread, but something we celebrate. Society reveres youth, and older people sometimes feel like their best years are behind them. They feel ignored and invisible. That's such a shame, because as you're about to discover, your best years lie ahead. Whether you're in your fifties, sixties, or even older, life can be exciting!

Hi, my name's Wendy and I'm seventy-two years old at the time of writing. My parents emigrated from the UK to a charming island called Mauritius in the early 1950s. I had a great early childhood playing with my friends in the mud and sun, among the free-range chickens and ducks. Hygiene was not something the locals considered especially important, and although Mum did her best with the only available disinfectant available; a bottle of 'Dettol', us kids used to get sick quite frequently. Little did I know, that was the best thing that could have happened for my long-term health. I developed a strong immune system.

When I was in my early sixties, I developed crippling back pain. X-rays showed it was caused by a prolapsed disc. From then on, I'm ashamed to admit, I let this chronic pain define me. I was low in energy, unable to sit for more than ten minutes at a time, unable to go out to dinner, or to even watch TV without lying on the floor. Walking was painful and my sleep was frequently interrupted.

I jumped on the merry-go-round of physiotherapy, chiropractic manipulation and remedial massage. *Nothing* worked. I tried orthopedic inserts in my shoes, special exercises from on-line back gurus and even hypnotherapy. I finally decided that this was my lot in life and decided to just put up with it. I was on heavy pain medication, which helped dull the pain, but it also dulled my senses.

Among all the doctors and so-called 'experts' I consulted, not *one* of them suggested it was my posture that could be to blame; that and too much sitting in front of the computer. I finally worked this out for myself, with the help of a long-term Facebook friend. I concentrated on correcting my posture, alternated sitting and standing during the day, practiced stretching and lifting my chest muscles and strengthening my core. After only two weeks, I noticed a huge improvement. After a few months, I was off all medication, and am now living a normal, pain-free life.

I simply tell you this story to illustrate that things can change for the better and that sometimes it's up to us to make that change ...

In the following chapters, I want to give people all the knowledge that I have accumulated over the years. I have a diploma in holistic health therapy and have a passion for natural health. As I've grown older, this has turned to an interest in healthy aging. What follows is what I have learned over the years of research and study of nutrition and how the body ages.

The diseases that are considered to be a natural part of aging, are not natural at all. We can all live a healthy, happy, and productive life into our nineties and beyond. I invite you to join me on this journey.

There's a lot of information within these pages and reading this book cover to cover may be likened to drinking from a firehose for some people. If that's you, feel free to start with the chapters that most concern you. However please read through the whole book if you can, as it will help your understanding of the material.

Chapter 2 – The Science of Aging

Telomeres – what are they and why should I care?

We each have our own unique DNA, as you would know if you read or watch crime thrillers on TV. But what is DNA and how does it affect the aging process?

DNA – short for *deoxyribonucleic acid* is a long, double-stranded molecule which contains twenty-three chromosomes. It's shaped like a circular twisted ladder. DNA contains our unique genetic blueprint and dictates characteristics like eye color, hair color, shape, and even intelligence levels, by transferring information within every cell in our body. DNA is passed down from one generation to another, the offspring having the combined DNA of both parents.

Telomeres are found at the ends of DNA strands to protect their chromosomes from fraying and becoming entangled, thus damaging the DNA, and therefore the cell itself. Cellular damage can lead to disease and a shorter lifespan. Each time a cell divides, the telomeres become shorter, until the cell cannot divide anymore and eventually dies.

Telomeres become shorter with age and it is now thought that the faster the telomeres shorten, the faster we age. So how can we delay the shortening of our telomeres?

Test tube studies have shown that telomeres shorten faster when exposed to oxidative stress. Oxidative stress is caused by *free radicals*, toxic by-products of oxygen metabolism. Free radicals act like rust in the body, causing damage to the cell membranes, leading to inflammation. In simple terms, the way to prevent telomere shortening is to do all we can to prevent oxidative stress, by taking antioxidants, eating a good diet, and avoiding the things that cause it. Smoking, chronic stress, junk food, obesity and some medications are a few of the triggers that can cause oxidative stress.

Telomere longevity is also increased by an enzyme called *telomerase*. Some scientists believe that increasing telomerase could be the simple answer to preserve telomere life. However, there is a flip side to this theory. Cancer cells also have telomeres, and tumor growth would also be enhanced by increasing telomerase. Cancer cells don't behave like normal cells. They subdivide much faster. A recent study has also associated increased risk of brain cancer with artificially increasing telomerase.

Research is still being done into telomeres, mainly to prevent genetic age-related disorders. Our DNA holds the secrets as to why people with certain genes develop cancer. There are still more questions than answers when it comes to our DNA. For now, the best natural ways that are thought to enhance telomerase production are exercise, intermittent fasting, meditation, probiotics, vitamin D, green tea, and antioxidant supplements (for example CoQ10 and curcumin).

We are not designed to live forever, but while we are here, we are entitled to live a happy disease-free life. This is the potential future of telomere research.

Sources:

http://www.faim.org/telomeres-major-discovery-reveals-the-secret-to-dramatically-slowing-aging
https://tmhome.com/benefits/study-tm-meditation-increase-telomerase/
http://articles.mercola.com/sites/articles/archive/2012/05/09/the-nutrients-most-likely-to-let-you-live-to-be-much-older-than-100.aspx
http://www.medicalnewstoday.com/articles/288515.php
https://www.nature.com/scitable/topicpage/introduction-what-is-dna-6579978
https://draxe.com/telomeres/
http://www.evergreennutrition.com/free-radicals-and-inflammation

https://well.blogs.nytimes.com/2010/01/27/phys-ed-how-exercising-keeps-your-cells-young/
https://draxe.com/top-10-high-antioxidant-foods/

Chapter 3 – Crawling Through the Maze of Diet Misinformation

"Vegetables are a must on a diet. I suggest carrot cake, zucchini bread, and pumpkin pie" - Jim Davis

Oh no! Now she's going to tell me what I can't eat ...

I will never tell you what to do; just advise and make you aware. So, let's start this chapter on a positive note. We'll look at all the delicious foods that are healthy too. Then we can slip in the nasty stuff after that.

Deal?

I remember one frustrated client asking me, *"Why is everything that tastes good, bad for me?"* I understand her frustration, and the answer is, we have been carefully groomed by 'Big Food'. There's so much salt and sugar added to processed foods and drinks, that our taste buds have become addicted.

It's a well-known fact that a diet high in vegetables is beneficial to our health, so there's no need to go over it at length here. There are other foods that enhance our health, that were previously given a bad name. However, they are perfectly safe to eat *in moderation*. For example:

Butter, eggs and cheese

These not only taste good but are good for you too. Surprised? These three foods come under the banner of 'saturated fats.

Saturated fat has long been touted as one of the 'bad' fats. It stems back from a flawed research study back in the 1950's by a man by the name of *Ancel Keys*. Mr. Keys published a paper that stated, dietary fat was the reason for the increase in heart disease in patients. More recent studies, taken over a larger slice of the population, has since disproved this. Still, over seventy years later, the myth persists.

Saturated fats are one of the few sources of vitamin K2, a vitamin that protects the heart. They also contain conjugated linoleic acid (CLA), stearic acid and palmitic acid. These have *no negative effect* on the heart and may even improve our immunity. Saturated fats are particularly good for our brain health.

So, enjoy butter in place of margarine and don't be afraid of eggs and cheese either. Over-consumption of saturated fats, or any fat, may lead to weight gain and other health problems, so enjoy them *in moderation.*

Coconut oil

This is a plant sourced, saturated fat that contains medium-chain fatty acids, an example of which is *lauric* acid. Lauric acid is an immune system booster. Coconut oil is one of the best oils for cooking as it has a high smoke point and doesn't break down over high heat.

Coconut milk

This makes a good substitute for cow's milk if you're sensitive to lactose. The milk of the coconut has similar properties to the oil.

Dark chocolate

If you're going to have a sugar fix, dark chocolate is a good choice. Choose one with 70% cocoa or higher. Dark chocolate is high in antioxidants and a few squares make a healthy treat.

Fruits

Yes, they're sweet and full of fructose. * So why are fruits healthy while sugar is not? There is a difference between the fructose in fruits and the sucrose in sugar. Fruits contain longer chain carbohydrates that take longer to digest and absorb. They also contain essential nutrients, antioxidants and fiber that are required for optimal digestion. Fruits are nature's sweet gifts. Enjoy them in moderation.

There is no similarity to the fructose in fruits to that in high fructose corn syrup.

Complex carbohydrates

These are the whole grain carbohydrates, whole wheat bread, oats, and certain vegetables to name a few. Complex carbohydrates contain fiber and other nutrients and are an important part of a healthy diet. There are groups of people who think carbohydrates, specifically grains, to be harmful to our bodies. I don't agree; however, I do respect these views.

While 'cutting carbs' may lead to short-term weight loss, it's never a good idea to cut out an entire macro food group from our diet for a long time.

Simple carbohydrates, on the other hand, offer little benefit. They have been stripped of their nutritional value and our bodies don't need them at all. Unfortunately, they are hard to avoid. For example, most processed foods contain either white flour or sugar.

Alternatives to white flour…

It's nice to enjoy a baked treat every now and again, but the vast majority of bakery goods are made with white flour. Here are some alternatives, rye flour, millet flour, almond meal, brown rice flour and oat flour.

Nuts

Nuts make healthy snacks, and the oils found in nuts are nutritious if kept fresh. Nuts are calorie dense, so if you're watching your weight, stick to a handful a day.

Super-foods

Some foods have been called super-foods due to their high nutritional value and ability to prevent disease. Here are a few examples:

Blueberries – Packed with vitamin C and fiber, blueberries contain powerful antioxidants (Anthocyanins). These lovely berries can lower blood pressure and lower LDL (bad) cholesterol. They're also credited with the potential to prevent certain cancers.

Broccoli – Possibly the best vegetable money can buy, broccoli is a member of the cruciferous family of vegetables. Broccoli contains fiber and a range of vitamins and minerals. Studies have shown a diet high in broccoli may prevent cancers – due to a compound called *sulforaphane*.

Quinoa – although it's a type of grain, quinoa is a protein packed super-food, which has the full range of amino acids, particularly *lysine*. Quinoa also contains magnesium, iron, and manganese.

Oatmeal – Perfect for those who are gluten intolerant, oatmeal is high in soluble fiber and can help lower cholesterol levels.

Spinach – It worked for Popeye, and it can benefit us too. Spinach is loaded with vitamins and minerals including zinc, which is an immune system booster. Unfortunately, spinach, especially the imported variety may be contaminated with DTD, so it's best to buy the organic spinach. Cook it lightly, or you'll end up with mush! Juicing is a great option for spinach. Just be aware; if you suffer from gout, spinach is high in purines, so eat it in moderation.

Coconut oil – The best oil for high heat cooking, due to its high *smoke point* (around 350 degrees F). Coconut oil has many health benefits (see the full explanation in the fats section below.)

Which foods should we avoid?

Sometimes, it's not what you cook, it's how you cook it.

Steaming is a great cooking method for vegetables, as it preserves the nutrients. However, it can get a tiny bit boring if we do it all the time.

One way to add pizzazz to our veggies is to stir-fry them. Roasting or grilling vegetables also brings out the natural flavor. Stir frying, roasting and grilling all use high temperatures so it's important to use an oil that will remain stable when exposed to high heat. This leads seamlessly into a discussion on…

Fats and oils.

Nowhere in all the mass of diet advice is there so much confusion as there is about good old FAT. A lot of people believe that fat is the enemy, especially when it comes to weight loss. But fat can be your friend.

There are many types of fats. Saturated, polyunsaturated, and monounsaturated.

In the era of the "fat free diet," which is thankfully losing popularity, all fats were considered evil. The only probable exception was Omega 3 which is an oil found in certain types of fish.

We've already spoken about saturated fats; butter, meat eggs, and how they're fine in moderation. So, what about polyunsaturated fats? Are they healthy? The answer is one that the lawyers love, "It depends".

There are some polyunsaturated fats which are essential to life, and some that can send us to an early grave. 'Good' polyunsaturated fats are Omega-3 oils from fish or Krill, flax-seed oil, oily nuts, such as walnuts or sunflower seeds, and green leafy vegetables.

The 'bad' Omega-3s include corn, soybean, safflower, and cottonseed oils. These are heavily refined and can trigger inflammation in the body. This in turn raises the body's production of cholesterol to cope with the inflammation. These refined oils form various harmful compounds when heated, such as *lipid peroxides* and *aldehydes*. Not only are these carcinogenic when eaten, they may vaporize and be inhaled into the lungs during cooking. Don't waste your money on these oils.

11

Monounsaturated fats

These include canola oil, peanut oil, high-oleic safflower oil, sesame oil and olive oil. Sesame oil has a strong flavor and is used in small amounts in Asian cuisine. Canola oil is a refined product of the rapeseed plant and is not recommended at all.

Olive oil - Extra virgin olive oil contains antioxidants and vitamin E, which help fight free radicals in the body. Using it for high heat cooking may destroy some of the nutrients and flavor. Refined olive oil has a higher smoke point than the extra virgin variety and is more suitable for frying and other high temperature cooking. Extra virgin olive oil is fine for normal cooking, however, and adds flavor and nutrients to the food.

Coconut oil – Formally scorned as unhealthy, as it contains saturated fat, coconut oil is finally getting the attention it deserves. In fact, coconut oil may belong to the top of the class when it comes to our health. It's used for cooking, and as a beauty aid for skin. Coconut oil's saturated fats are not the same as those found in animal fats. They're *medium chain triglycerides* or MCTs. Fifty percent of these MCTs is *lauric acid* which can destroy harmful toxins like bacteria, viruses, and fungi. Lauric acid is good for diabetics as it doesn't raise insulin levels when consumed.

Therefore, it's not necessary to limit the quantity of coconut oil we consume. MCTs are metabolized differently in our bodies. After digestion, they are sent to the liver, where they are used either as a source of energy or turned into ketones, which can have therapeutic effects on brain disorders like Alzheimer's.

Coconut oil can also help us lose weight, as it keeps us feeling fuller for longer, thus reducing appetite. It also helps reduce cholesterol levels in the blood. Some tropical countries rely on the coconut as their main food staple, and their health has not suffered for it.

Trans fats ☹

Most everyone knows about trans fats these days, due to their negative publicity. Trans fats are artificially manufactured by a process known as *hydrogenation*. This involves passing hydrogen gas through heated vegetable oil. From there, a solvent is added (typically *hexane*) and the product is then deodorized and bleached.

Why would anyone go to all that trouble? Because it produces a stable source of fat which is cheap and doesn't break down. Products made with trans fats last longer on the shelves. Food manufacturers fell in love with trans fats, and they spread rapidly into the food industry. There was one small inconvenience, however. Heart disease spread rapidly through the population. Despite this, it seems Big Food is more interested in their bottom line than our health. Imagine!

How to avoid trans fats -

These artificial fats are found mainly in refined vegetable oils, margarine, processed foods like crackers, potato chips and biscuits, and deep-fried foods. Trans fats have no nutritional value and raise the risk of inflammation, clogged arteries, type 2 diabetes, and heart disease. Even bottles of healthy oil, for example olive oil, can contain trans fats, if the manufacturer has combined different oils together. Check the label for trans fats, or *hydrogenated vegetable oil* (trans fat in disguise)

Not all trans fats are bad -

There are such things as healthy natural trans fats. These are naturally occurring trans fats from cattle and other animals that naturally graze on grass (grass fed). These natural trans fats contain conjugated linoleic acid (CLA) and can help in muscle building and even weight loss. If the animals have been fed on grains, these natural trans fats are of a much lower quality.

Bear in mind, the trans fats used in processed foods are most likely to be the artificially produced fats. Although declaring trans fats on food labels in some countries is mandatory, it isn't in others. Always check that label. *There is no safe level of trans fats.*

Fats can be awfully complicated! To keep it simple, use coconut and olive oil for cooking and olive oil on your salad. Enjoy small amounts of butter and cheese in your diet and you can't go wrong.

Refined carbohydrates (White rice, white flour, white just about anything else...)

Refined carbohydrates are those that have been modified and stripped of nutritional value. They have now taken over the blame from fats, for the huge rise of obesity and chronic disease in our population. White flour, pasta, white rice, and sugar are the main culprits.

White flour is a simple carbohydrate, made from wheat, which has had all its nutritional value stripped out. Enriched white flour has had extra vitamins added to it. Whole wheat, whole grain, or whole meal flour still contains the wheat germ, endosperm, and husk. It's a much better option. Whole meal pasta is also available in the health section of most supermarkets.

White flour is everywhere. There are products that contain flour that you might not have even considered. For example, thickeners in gravies and sauces. Products made with whole grain flour are simply much better but be aware that some "brown" breads just contain coloring, not whole meal flour.

Sugar

Most people think sugar is bad because it causes weight gain and contributes to tooth decay, but it goes further than that. Sugar is the worst of the refined carbohydrates. It's calorie dense and contains no nutritional value at all. Eating a diet high in sugar can cause insulin resistance and lead to diabetes and liver disease. Over consumption of sugar causes inflammation in the body and can raise cholesterol levels.

Cancer cells love sugar too. If you have a high cancer risk, avoid sugar as much as possible. Sugar is in most processed foods, even savory foods such as tomato ketchup, baked beans, some Chinese food, bread, and coleslaw dressing. Even eating simple carbohydrates, like a slice of white bread, will raise glucose (sugar) levels in the blood. Simple carbohydrates convert to glucose very quickly as part of the digestion process.

Unfortunately, sugar is an extremely addictive food and requires considerable willpower to give up. In fact, it's so addictive, it's been referred to as a drug by some nutritionists.

If you want some help giving up sugar, we had a fun 5-day challenge that I've converted into a free workshop. People have found this extremely helpful for cutting down their sugar consumption. Simply login to register here: **https://ageinreverse.com.au/courses/how-to-stop-annoying-sugar-cravings-in-5-days/**

There are natural alternatives to sugar such as Stevia and Xylitol. Stevia is an herbal plant that has a long-lasting aftertaste and can take some getting used to. Xylitol has around 40% of the calories of sugar and is made from wood bark. It also tastes a lot like the real thing. However, it can cause stomach upsets in some people.

Chemical sweeteners are not a viable alternative and can cause many health problems. *Aspartame* is particularly deadly. Aspartame appears as *NutraSweet, Equal, Spoonful* etc. Why is this product so harmful, particularly for those who are trying to lose weight?

After a lengthy delay, due to health concerns from several scientists, the FDA approved aspartame for general use in 1996, mostly due to pressure from the food giant, *Monsanto*. Aspartame contains ingredients (aspartate and glutamate) that act as neurotransmitters in the brain. These ingredients can kill brain neurons by generating free radicals. The *Federation of American Societies for Experimental Biology* (FASEB) has issued a warning to women of childbearing age to stop using aspartame, due to the risk to the fetus. Add to that, children, the elderly, and those with chronic diseases, and you have a good slice of the population.

Many people who want to lose weight turn to artificial sweeteners because they're zero-calorie sweeteners. Aspartame, for instance, is 200 times sweeter than sugar. While this is not a problem in itself, aspartame does not activate the food rewards pathways in the brain, whereas eating sugar does. Therefore, your appetite is not sated and you'll want to eat more.

Anything that tastes sweet increases appetite, no matter what is used sweeten the food. Repeated exposure to sweet foods and drinks encourages a greater craving for them.

Following are just *some* of the side effects of aspartame, weight gain, heart palpitations, migraines, anxiety, tinnitus, depression, memory loss, irritability and fatigue.

At the end of the day, the best way to avoid sugar and most other unhealthy ingredients is to avoid highly processed foods and select whole, natural, non-processed foods instead. I know time is a problem; there's never enough time to cook meals from scratch. Instead, try reframing this. Think about the years you'll be adding to your life by doing this one simple thing every day.

It's not easy to change our eating habits, so why not do it gradually? Every week take one harmful ingredient from your diet and replace it with a better one. In a couple of months, you'll feel healthier and happier!

Sources:

http://www.healthline.com/nutrition/5-studies-on-saturated-fat#section1

http://www.medicalnewstoday.com/articles/266765.php

http://foodfacts.mercola.com/spinach.html

https://authoritynutrition.com/is-olive-oil-good-for-cooking/

http://healthyeating.sfgate.com/wholegrain-pasta-vs-regular-pasta-3476.html

https://authoritynutrition.com/top-10-evidence-based-health-benefits-of-coconut-oil/

http://www.livestrong.com/article/336585-list-of-no-white-flour-foods/

http://www.livestrong.com/article/34752-stop-eating-sugar-flour/

http://articles.mercola.com/sites/articles/archive/2011/11/06/aspartame-most-dangerous-substance-added-to-food.aspx

http://articles.mercola.com/sites/articles/archive/2016/12/06/aspartame-causes-obesity.aspx

https://www.globalhealingcenter.com/natural-health/aspartame-makes-you-gain-weight/

https://draxe.com/monounsaturated-fat/

http://articles.mercola.com/sites/articles/archive/2010/10/22/coconut-oil-and-saturated-fats-can-make-you-healthy.aspx

Chapter 4 - Exercise

"Whenever I feel like exercise, I lie down until the feeling passes." - *Robert M. Hutchins*

Exercise is nature's Prozac. Exercise manufactures chemicals called *endorphins*, in the brain; some examples being serotonin, testosterone and human growth hormone (HGH). Serotonin can enhance mood and reduce pain. It can take from ten to thirty minutes of exercise, depending on the individual, but once you've felt it, you won't want to stop. This is the reason why some people get "hooked" on exercise.

"…But I hate exercise…" If I had a penny for each time I've heard that, I'd be wealthy today. Exercise is what our bodies were built for; it improves our health in so many ways. Exercise keeps us slim, prevents disease, makes us happier, builds muscles and bones, builds confidence, improves balance, reduces stress, improves sleep, improves flexibility, prevents osteoporosis, improves our skin, and makes us feel so much better in every way. And if that's not enough, it adds years to our lifespan.

How to enjoy exercise

Start *slowwwly*.

Set yourself a goal, even if it's just a five-minute walk. Most of us can tolerate the idea of five minutes. If it's raining, or too hot/cold/windy, just walk around the house, or around a shopping mall. If you can do that, you'll probably find yourself walking further over time. Walking will become a habit and you'll feel like something's missing if you don't do it. You'll find a way to fit it into your day, no matter what.

Buy an exercise DVD, or an online exercise program. It makes you feel like you're not doing it alone, and you'll enjoy moving to the music while saving on those expensive gym fees. There's no need to ever set foot in a gym unless you want to. I have a few programs that I use often. I buy my weights from Kmart, and I try to gradually increase them over time.

Some people find that group classes motivate them. This is a great way to get moving and make new friends too.

Find something you enjoy and just do it. Here's some motivational videos to get you going:

https://www.youtube.com/watch?v=HSbmO7nn_4M

https://www.youtube.com/watch?v=L3iLPrkIr9E

https://www.youtube.com/watch?v=mhU0X3uYA14

Now that you're moving, there are 3 main types of exercise:

Aerobic – Walking, running, cycling etc. Good for general health.

Resistance - This strengthens the muscles and bones. Weightlifting or bodyweight exercises fit into this category.

Flexibility – This is *super* beneficial for older people. It's basically stretching. This can make us feel younger and suits any fitness level. It prevents injury during physical activity.

If you can fit all three types into your weekly routine, you'll really feel the benefit. Of course, you don't have to do them all every day.

There is one particular type of exercise which dramatically speeds up weight loss if that's your goal. You'll need to build up a reasonable level of fitness first though, otherwise it can put too much stress on your heart.

It's called *high intensity interval training* (HIIT), and combines a period of slow movement, followed by very rapid movement. This can be done by walking and running, riding a bike slowly then much faster, or even swimming at different speeds. Start with three minutes of slow movement followed by one minute of going as fast as you can. There are programs you can buy online that show you how to do that, but you don't need fancy moves. YouTube has free videos you can search for, or simply doing the above works just as well. Simply increase the times and intensity as your fitness improves.

The one, and maybe the only thing, you will need is a good pair of walking/running shoes, with good arch support. Chose a comfortable pair that come far enough up the back of the heel, so they grip your foot well.

Aerobic exercise – this can be as gentle or as intense as you need it to be. If you're very unfit, start with a slow walk. Slowly increase the speed and distance as you start to feel fitter. Once you're walking fast for thirty minutes or longer and are not out of breath, add some hills to your walk. When you reach this level, you'll be feeling and looking a lot better. I used to jog but stopped when I was in my fifties. Running is hard on the knee joints, and you don't need to run to get fit, unless you really love running. Walking is equally beneficial; it just takes longer.

Aerobic exercise will keep the heart and lungs working well and will stimulate the lymphatic system to remove toxins from the body. You can work aerobics into your day. Mowing the lawn, walking upstairs, line dancing or walking the dog.

Resistance exercise – You don't have to buy weights when starting out; anything can be used as a weight. You can even use your own body as a weight. Space limits me from putting exercise diagrams here, but there are some good resources on YouTube for bodyweight exercises in the sources below. Always keep your tummy muscles firm when doing resistance exercise, to protect your spine. This is especially important when lifting weights above your head. Some yoga or Pilates moves use the body's weight and doing these can have the same strengthening effect as lifting weights. Resistance exercise will strengthen bones and muscles and make your whole body stronger.

Flexibility exercise – Stretching can prevent aches and pains, make you taller, increase your range of motion and improve posture. If we don't stretch, our muscles shrink and become tight. This is especially important if you sit for extended periods each day. Stretching was the way I moved myself out of chronic pain a few months ago. I was walking, doing yoga and Pilates and lifting correctly, but nothing helped, until I started stretching. Try this; lift your chest upwards and pull your shoulders down and back, pulling your head back gently. If your posture is poor, you'll feel uncomfortable at first. Keep doing this until it's a habit. You'll add inches to your height and that niggling back pain might just start to improve.

Which muscles should you stretch? The most important are the shoulders and front of chest, calves, hamstrings, hip flexors and the quadriceps (front of the thighs). If you have chronic pain, do this every day after warming up with a short walk. Otherwise, three to four times a week is fine.

I really hope this has given you the motivation to start exercising. In my opinion, exercise is second only to breathing, eating, and drinking. Can you exercise too much? Of course. Too much of anything is harmful. You'll learn how much exercise is ideal for you, as you progress.

Sources:

https://greatist.com/fitness/50-bodyweight-exercises-you-can-do-anywhere

http://www.health.harvard.edu/staying-healthy/the-importance-of-stretching

https://www.exercise.com/blog/how-much-exercise-is-necessary-for-endorphin-release/

https://www.healthdirect.gov.au/physical-activity-guidelines-for-older-adults

Chapter 5 - Alternative Healing Systems

"The art of healing comes from nature, not from the physician. Therefore, the physician must start from nature, with an open mind" - Paracelsus

Energy medicine, or energy therapy, is fast becoming a popular way of reducing stress and anxiety, easing chronic pain, losing weight, giving up smoking, and dealing with food cravings. In this chapter, I'm including two different types of energy therapy. They're both free to use, and extremely effective; I've used them myself many times and am still amazed how such simple practices can work so well. Even if you're skeptical about this type of healing protocol, I urge you to try it, as it will work, whether or not you believe in it.

Percussion Suggestion Technique

The first energy technique is called, PSTEC, or *Percussion Suggestion Technique*. PSTEC is a technique for positive, personal change. It can remove negative thoughts and emotions, relieve physical pain, calm anxiety, accelerate weight loss, promote self-confidence, and be used for a host of other issues. The audio tracks for removing emotional distress are free. Their main website can be found here - https://www.pstec.org/.

PSTEC may be one of the best ways to access the sub-conscious mind; the place where our deepest beliefs about ourselves exist. Some of these beliefs, and the emotions they create, are harmful to our health and wellbeing. The sub-conscious mind is extremely powerful, much more so than the conscious mind. The trouble is, we can't access it directly and have no way of knowing what negative beliefs lie within. The subconscious mind controls *all* our emotions, beliefs, and behaviors.

PSTEC can access this hidden mind and erase our negative beliefs, setting us free to pursue a more healthy and prosperous life. I have used it on myself and on clients for all sorts of issues.

The creator of PSTEC, Tim Phizackerley – don't try to say it with your mouth full – has many qualifications, including, Diploma with Distinction in Clinical Hypnotherapy, Bachelor of Education Honors Degree, and has featured many times on British radio as an expert on personal change. Tim started out as a hypnotherapist, finally creating PSTEC to help those with particularly difficult issues, such as anorexia and bulimia. Using his past background in computer programming, Tim created a series of audio tracks, which have now expanded to include many other personal issues. Among these are relationship problems, post-traumatic stress, self-esteem, phobias, nicotine addiction, and even abundance issues around money.

PSTEC can be described as an alternative to cognitive behavior therapy, NLP or hypnotherapy. It's mainly used as a self-help tool, although many practitioners are now including it in their arsenal to help people with a multitude of physical and mental health problems, confidence problems, weight loss, chronic pain, and money issues.

The link below is to a video that shows how everyday people are achieving incredible results with PSTEC.

https://www.pstec.org/talks.php

Here is the link to other free resources:

https://www.pstec.org/free-therapy-resources.php

N.B – The audio tracks to remove negative beliefs are not free, but the free tracks should be used first.

Eutaptics©

The second technique is called Eutaptics©, previously known as *Faster EFT*. It was created by Robert G Smith, a personal growth expert, after many years of testing research and experimentation.

Eutaptics© has evolved from the original EFT (Emotional Freedom Technique) which is an energy-based therapy. Eutaptics© is a blend of NLP (Neuro Linguistic Programming), BSFF (Be Set Free Fast), acupressure, psychology, all mixed together with a sprinkling of spirituality. Eutaptics© takes the best of these modalities and combines them together into a powerful healing system.

Eutaptics© is a self-help protocol that is very simple to use. It is based on the premise that the mind and body are not separate but operate together to create the whole being. Therefore the mind has the ability to heal the body.

It can work on various conditions, such as chronic pain, depression, post-traumatic stress disorder (PTSD), addictions, body dysmorphia and negative beliefs to name just a few. And yes, it works even if you're skeptical and think it's a lot of 'hocus-pocus'! This modality has changed many peoples' lives for the better and has a loyal following of people whose lives have been transformed, simply by using this simple technique. Many of these have gone on to become Eutaptics© practitioners, treating others and spreading the word.

If I had to explain how Eutaptics© works in one sentence, I would say that it neutralizes painful memories, emotions, and experiences, into more positive ones. It does this by a clever 'pattern interrupt' process.

The basic technique of Eutaptics©

First, focus on the problem at hand; it can be anything that's bothering you in the current moment. Give the problem a point score from one to ten; with one being a non-issue and 10 being a profoundly serious and disturbing one. This is called the SUDS, or *subjective units of distress scale*. Then ask yourself, "How do you know that you have the

24

problem?" It may be a feeling of distress, chronic pain or simply a feeling of discomfort in the solar plexus, stomach, or throat.

After that, let the feeling go and concentrate on the sensation of your fingers tapping on your skin. Simply tap on the following points while saying, "Release and let it go":

1.   Eyebrow point – top inner edge of the eyebrow, near the bridge of the nose.

2.   Side of eye point - the outer side of the eye, just below the temple.

3.   Under eye point – the bony area just under the eye.

4.   Collar bone point – under the collarbone, off center of the chest

After doing this, simply circle your wrist with your other hand, take a deep breath and focus on a pleasant memory. Then breathe out while saying, "Peace."

There's no need to tap hard, and you can use either hand or both hands for this process. It really helps to have a pleasant memory in mind before you start. It could be a peaceful sunset over the ocean, a beautiful garden, a cute puppy, or anything else that makes you feel relaxed and at peace.

After doing the above, check back with your problem; chances are it will have shifted slightly. Do you feel better? If so re-evaluate your score. What started out as a ten, may now have gone down to a five. If not repeat the process until the problem seems insignificant.

Here's a YouTube video that shows the basic tapping protocol of Eutaptics© (Faster EFT). It's an older video, but the principals still apply - https://www.youtube.com/watch?v=UnTwiQY2hcM

What I've outlined above, is a simplified version of Eutaptics©. There are issues you may have that are more complex; maybe caused by beliefs instilled in you when you were a child. These issues may take a lot longer and have many associated memories, emotions, and false, negative beliefs. They may take days or even weeks to fully tap out. You may not even feel any different during the first few rounds of tapping.

Many people are tempted to give up at this stage, but if you persevere and tap on the issue every day, eventually you *will* get a result. If you have severe emotional problems, for example PTSD, there are experts who are especially trained to deal with these. Contacting a Eutaptics© professional may be the best way forward for you. You can meet with them directly or have a session via phone, Skype, or even live video, in some cases.

Sources:

https://www.besetfreefast.com/bsff-for-beginners

http://www.pstec.org/

https://eutaptics.org/

https://stressexpert.com/7-ways-eutaptics-different-eft/

https://robertgene.com/

Section 2 - The Diseases of Aging

Disclaimer - The information in these chapters is not intended to replace a one-on-one relationship with a qualified health care professional, neither is it intended as medical advice. You are advised to consult your medical practitioner.

(New chapter added August 2020) A lot of people have asked me about the immune system and why older people are more at risk from new diseases. I have added this chapter below.

Chapter 6 – Age and the Immune System

Our immune system is not one single organ, it's a series of systems throughout the body. This system is loosely divided into two parts, the *innate* and *adaptive.*

The innate immune system is our first line of defense. It consists mainly of the skin, the mucus membranes in the nose and throat and chemicals in the blood. The innate immune system responds quickly to any invading antigens (bacteria, fungi, and viruses) that invade the body, sending white blood cells in a complex procedure to stop infection.

The adaptive immune system has *acquired immunity*, meaning it can identify a specific pathogen (germ) that it has previously encountered. This is how immunity is built from childhood, and why young children seems to always come home from school with various types of health issues. They are encountering new germs and haven't yet built up their adaptive immunity.

As they grow into adulthood, this immunity build up until it can identify various pathogens, like the common cold and some strains of flu. Unfortunately, these pathogens keep mutating, which is why a large number of people come down with these diseases each year. However these adults are unlikely to contract measles, mumps, or chicken pox, as they have already had these diseases and have produced the antibodies, or they have been vaccinated against them.

Why do older adults have weaker immunity?

Given the above, you would think that the older we get, the better our immune systems should work, and in some ways they do. The problem arises when an older person encounters a *new* pathogen that the immune system cannot recognize. This cuts out adaptive immunity function and puts all the stress of the innate immune system.

The typical line of thought is that the immune system slows down, along with a lot of other bodily functions, as we age. The older person's immune system is not as robust as a younger person's. Not only do we have fewer immune cells, but the ones we have are weakened and don't communicate with each other as efficiently. Their reaction time has slowed, which gives pathogens more time to enter the body and wreak havoc.

However this has never been proven and there is a new line of thought that older people succumb to diseases, not because their immune systems are weaker, but because they're actually working too hard. However this is just a theory for now.

Add to this, some older individuals have other health problems, such as type 2 diabetes and low-grade chronic inflammation which weaken the immune system, and the cause becomes largely irrelevant. What is encouraging, is that the healthier we are, the better our immune response will be, at any age.

The immune response is extraordinarily complex, and this chapter may have oversimplified it, but I hope you get the idea of how it works. The important thing is how do we keep our immune systems as strong as they can be?

The best and only way is to improve your health. Specifically:

- Keep your stress levels down by tapping or deep breathing

- Get plenty of sleep. This will tend to happen when your stress improves

- Cut down on processed food

- Move more. Don't worry if you can't achieve 10,000 steps, just increase your movement

- Get into nature. This is called 'forest bathing' and it has great health benefits

When you feel stronger, this increases your confidence and gets you out of the fear state.

Sources

https://health.usnews.com/health-care/patient-advice/articles/2018-03-14/how-aging-affects-your-immune-system

https://www.webmd.com/healthy-aging/guide/seniors-boost-immunity#1

https://www.ncbi.nlm.nih.gov/pmc/articles/PMC5291468/

Chapter 7 - Cancer

"Cancer is a Word, not a Sentence." - Robert Buckman

A cancer diagnosis is scary, but the survival rate is improving. Cancer patients have more control over the disease these days than ever. This is partly due to improved medical treatments and better doctor/patient communication, but mainly because people are becoming more aware of natural health and how they can influence their body's response to disease.

Most people instinctively know that the body comes with the ability to heal itself. I'm not suggesting for one moment that anyone should decide to take on cancer by themselves. Can a cancer patient heal themselves? Yes, but it makes much more sense to take advantage of medical science and find out what it has to offer.

We all know about the side effects of chemotherapy and radiation. These treatments do kill cancer cells, but they also affect healthy cells and have a devastating effect on the immune system, which is our main defense against cancer. This is the main problem from my point of view.

At the time of writing, new research is being done into safer types of chemotherapy and less traumatic cancer cures. It's worth finding out the latest information from your doctor.

But a small percentage of people do take notice. They listen, they think … and they change.

Which one are you?

Cancer is a wakeup call. It holds a mirror up to your life. Can you look into that mirror? Are you courageous enough? Not everyone that is diagnosed with cancer has brought on the disease, but some have. If you can acknowledge that a lifestyle choice may have been the cause of your cancer, then you have a lot of courage and your recovery rate will improve. You have taken responsibility for your health. And that's a wonderful achievement!

We all have cancer cells in our bodies. A normal, healthy immune system will remove most of these. The immune system is our first line of defense. The stronger your immune system is, the lower the chance of developing cancer.

What is cancer? It's a group of rogue cells with damaged DNA, that multiply rapidly. Cancer is a symptom of a sick body, and an immune system that's so overloaded with toxic waste and starved of nutrients, that it has reached a tipping point.

However, even at this stage the body is programed to self-heal. It attempts to do this by building a barrier around the cancer cells. This is what we call a tumor. Removing the tumor can remove the cancer cells; the symptom has been removed. The cause, however, remains …

What causes cancer?

There are many things that can cause cancer. We are swimming in a sea of chemicals these days. Each day, many tons of chemicals are produced in factories around the world. These chemicals leak into the air, the water supply and even our food supply, due to pesticides and chemical fertilizers.

To add to the chemical soup, we use skincare, deodorants and air fresheners made from chemicals. Why not? They're available everywhere; they're cheap and they smell nice too.

We eat convenience food because there's never enough time to cook. We're stressed over our finances, our kids, our jobs, and our relationships. We fall asleep at our desks and lay awake in our beds. It's all just part of modern life. But the stress causes inflammation, and inflammation puts a huge load on our immune systems. Stress releases cortisol which depresses the immune system, as does negativity and hostility.

Add to this, EMFs (electromagnetic fields) from our phones and WIFI, toxic poisoning from heavy metals such as mercury and lead, fake estrogen or *xeno estrogen*, chemical hormones from birth control and menopause treatments, and it's a wonder that we are still here! Even babies are born, these days, with over 200 chemicals in their bloodstream.

But our immune systems are powerful and they can ward off most of the damage, even from things they were never designed for. So enough of the negativity and histrionics; lets concentrate on healing the damage and making ourselves as healthy as we can be!

Most doctors are well-meaning individuals. But they are trained in universities funded by the pharmaceutical companies. Doctors are given minimal training in subjects like nutrition, and none at all in natural health. Doctors are trained to heal sickness, not to promote wellness. Which means…

We need to take responsibility for our own health. Yes I'm being repetitive!

To strengthen our immune systems so they can best deal with diseases such as cancer, we need to expel as many toxins from our bodies as possible. Our bodies do a reasonable job of this on their own. They eliminate waste via the liver and kidneys, through our skin and lymphatic system, through breathing and defecation. But our bodies were never designed to cope with life in the twenty first century, and all the man-made toxins we are now exposed to.

What exactly are toxins? Toxins are substances that are poisonous to the body. They come from mold, pesticides, polluted air and water, car exhaust fumes and chemicals in personal products, just to name a few.

Heavy metals, such as fluoride, mercury, uranium, bromine, and chlorine are toxic as they can deplete our bodies of healthy minerals. For instance, mercury can replace zinc, as it uses the same cell receptors. Bromine, fluoride, and chlorine can replace iodine. Zinc boosts immunity and iodine is needed to metabolize food into energy, and for optimal thyroid function.

How to remove toxins from the body

Certain foods can remove toxins. Plant foods do this best, as they contain fiber that can capture toxic material and help eliminate it. Strawberries have a type of fiber that is not dissolved by stomach acid, and can bind with mercury and remove it. Quinoa can also help remove mercury. Spirulina and Chlorella will help remove uranium. Fruit seeds absorb arsenic. Modified Citrus Pectin – available in health stores – is also useful in removing heavy metals from the body.

Coffee is not that healthy when consumed, yet coffee *enemas* can remove a huge amount of toxins and strengthen the liver, which struggles to clean the blood of toxic waste.

If a body is overwhelmed by toxins, chelation therapy may be the best option.

Earth is our best doctor. Food is our best medicine. Plant foods, fresh from the soil will strengthen immunity. Vegetables are a rich source of Phyto-nutrients, enzymes, vitamins, minerals, and fiber. Vegetables, eaten whole or juiced, can prevent the acid environment in which cancer cells thrive. The body has a narrow range of acid/alkaline balance of 7.35 - 7.45 and will do everything it can to maintain that. It will attempt to rid itself of acid through breathing and sweating. As a last resort, it will extract minerals from our bones, cells and tissues in a bid to maintain alkaline levels, causing weakening of the bones.

To prevent this, make sure you maintain levels of these essential mineral by supplementing with minerals such as calcium, magnesium, sodium, and potassium. Calcium is best taken with vitamin D3 and vitamin K2 which ensure proper absorption and prevents calcium deposits from clogging the arteries.

There are those who advocate alkaline water to control acid levels, but this has not been scientifically proven. Too much alkalinity can be as dangerous as too much acidity. It's safer to eat natural alkaline foods such as vegetables. Buy organic if you can afford to; if not, grow your own. If that's not an option, at least know this - vegetables that form under the soil (carrots, turnips, beetroots) are less subject to toxic pesticides than those that grow above it (spinach, corn, broccoli etc.). Sprouting from vegetable seeds is always a good option, as sprouts contain higher amounts of enzymes.

Stay away from GMO (Genetically Modified Organism) foods - sometimes amusingly referred to as *frankenfoods*. They have altered DNA, and the long-term effects on our anatomy is not yet known. However, if man has tampered with them, it's not likely to be good.

Having removed the toxins from the body, we need to make sure we're getting the right nutrition into it, to strengthen our immunity. Refer to the chapter on diet, for a complete breakdown on the best foods to eat for optimal health. An anti-cancer diet is also a weight loss diet, without the need for resorting to fad diets, shakes etc.

Natural Cures for Cancer

Natural doctors believe that cancer cannot develop or thrive in an oxygen rich environment. Cancer also dislikes environments that are alkaline. So, we must prepare our terrain by removing stress, toxins, and acid waste. Then we stimulate our immune system by giving it the nutrition it needs.

This will bring down inflammation and dramatically reduce our risk of, not only cancer, but other diseases as well. A healthy immune system may also lessen our chance of developing auto-immune diseases, such as rheumatoid arthritis and lupus.

Google "natural cures for cancer", and you will find an alarming array of different 'cures' for cancer, ranging from exotic plants to laughter therapy. Do they work? Probably some do for some people, mainly because the patient believes that they will. Hence the placebo effect takes over, and the person's own mind heals their body.

Obviously, there are a lot of 'quack' cures out there, and a lot of people falsely claiming to be able to cure cancer. However, there are natural cures that carry some weight of proof, and it's those that we are most interested in. For those who want to go down the chemotherapy or radiation treatment route, these natural cures can make the journey easier and promote faster healing. Seek medical advice before doing this, of course.

Probiotics – Also known as "good" bacteria, these are microorganisms which can balance your intestinal microflora. You can eat probiotic food or take probiotic supplements. Best food sources are, kefir, yogurt, sauerkraut, and other fermented foods. Agricultural procedures like soaking produce in chlorine, can kill probiotics. Processed foods contain little to none.

I recommend supplements if you are fighting, or want to prevent, cancer. Around 80% of our immune system is housed in our digestive system. Probiotics can increase our immunity by improving food absorption, healing leaky gut, skin problems, chronic fatigue, joint pain, and many other health issues. In fact, probiotics can benefit every system in our body. Do the research and look for high quality brands with a high CFU *(colony forming units)* count and a high number of different strains of probiotic. These should be kept refrigerated.

Coffee Enemas – An extremely effective detoxication routine. As recommended in the *Gerson Method*, coffee enemas can double the rate of the flow of lymphatic fluid. This allows the lymphatic system to dispose of toxins much faster. Coffee enemas are particularly good at detoxifying the liver, while also cleansing the colon of built up waste. The alkalinity of the tissues is a direct result. While coffee enemas can be done at home; you can buy a kit for this purpose, I could think of nothing worse! It's extremely messy and there could be a risk of perforating the bowel. Leave it to those who know what they're doing.

Proteolytic Enzyme Therapy – Enzymes have been used as a treatment for cancer for over one hundred years. Yes, those old doctors knew a thing or two, and, more importantly, were able to practice their knowledge without fear of persecution. Proteolytic enzymes are similar to the *pancreatic enzymes*, naturally produced by the pancreas. They can reduce inflammation, and thus heal a multitude of bodily ills.

How do proteolytic enzymes work? Enzymes are needed for proper food digestion. Proteolytic enzymes help digest protein foods, such as meat, into amino acids. Undigested food can cause inflammation and leaky gut. Proteolytic enzymes also circulate in the blood and can detect cancer stem cells that the immune system cannot identify, due to their protective layer of protein. The enzymes strip the protein allowing the detection and destruction of these cancer cells by the immune system.

While the pancreas *does* produce enzymes, this process slows with age. Our bodies also rely on the foods we eat to have sufficient enzymes for their own digestion. Diets full of processed foods have all the enzymes removed. Changing to a fresh, or raw food diet can significantly raise enzyme consumption. Pineapple and papaya are two of the best food sources. Others are kiwi fruit, sauerkraut, yogurt, and kefir. *Note - the last three examples also contain probiotics.*

Stomach acid can destroy proteolytic enzymes, so it's best to look for supplements that are *"enteric-coated"*. This will prevent the tablet from being broken down in the stomach. An enteric-coated tablet passes safely into the small intestine, where the enzymes are best utilized.

Taking enzymes with food, helps in the digestion of that food. Taking them *between* meals, allow enzymes passage into the bloodstream where they can be used systemically.

Proteolytic enzymes don't have significant side effects, but can increase bleeding, so are not recommended a few days before or after surgery.

Vitamin C Chelation – We touched on chelation above. Chelation is a chemical reaction and can be carried out orally or intravenously. Vitamin C is one of the most important vitamins to support immune health. Humans, unlike most other animals, don't have the capacity to manufacture vitamin C, so it must come from our food, or from supplements. As an anti-oxidant and immune booster, vitamin C is crucial in the fight against cancer (particularly colorectal cancer), as suggested by Dr. Linus Pauling in the 1950s. Foods high in vitamin C include citrus fruits, berries, pineapple, kiwi-fruit, mango, kale, chili and bell peppers (capsicum), broccoli, papaya and cauliflower. Don't cook the life out of these, as vitamin C is destroyed at high temperatures. If taking supplements, make sure to choose those that include bioflavonoids.

When fighting cancer, intravenous vitamin C can induce oxidative damage to cancer cells, increasing the rate of die-off through the increased levels of hydrogen peroxide. Vitamin C taken orally is not capable of doing this, although it does have definite health benefits.

Vitamin D3 – Vitamin D3 is actually a hormone that is typically recommended for bone health. Recent research has found that vitamin D3 may also be a powerful way to prevent cancer. Research is ongoing, however a 2007 controlled double blind clinical trial had some positive results. This trial involved over a thousand post-menopausal women over a period of four years. It measured a 1400-1500 milligram supplement of calcium on its own, compared to the calcium with an added 1,100 IU of vitamin D3. Results after only 12 months showed the risk of cancer had decreased by almost 80% in the calcium + vitamin D group.

Vitamin D3 is available as a supplement and can form naturally in the human body on exposure to sunlight. As it is an oil soluble vitamin, it's best not to exceed 5,000 IU in supplement form. Take this vitamin with foods that include fat for best results. Make sure to take the D3 form and not the chemically produced vitamin D2, which is much less effective.

Curcumin – Curcumin is a spice which has antioxidant and anti-inflammatory properties. Laboratory studies have found curcumin to have anti-cancer effects, including development, growth and spread of the disease. Used in conjunction with chemotherapy, it promotes faster healing, particularly from breast, stomach, bowel, and skin cancers.

Oxygen Therapy – Whereas a normal healthy cell thrives on oxygen, cancer cells are different. They can live an in anaerobic environment (without oxygen) but require a large amount of glucose to survive. According to Dr. Otto Warburg, MD, lack of oxygen is a leading cause of cancer, and oxygen therapy is a safe and natural way to kill cancer cells. Dr. Warburg won the Nobel prize for Physiology in 1931, so it can be assumed he knew what he was talking about. Those were the days before Big Pharma had come upon the scene.

Getting more oxygen into the body is not something that we can do at home unfortunately. It involves the use of a *Hyperbaric Chamber*. Although not yet completely accepted by mainstream medicine, some hospitals have invested in these units and are using them to treat patients. A Hyperbaric Chamber creates air pressure which is about 2.5 times greater than normal. This allows the blood to absorb a greater amount of oxygen, which is transported to the body's cells and tissues. Aside from cancer, oxygen therapy is thought to cure other health problems as well.

Oxygen therapy is practiced worldwide and is relatively safe when done properly. Consult the International *Oxidative Medicine Association* (IOMA) to find a practitioner in your part of the world.

What options do we have today?

Because health funds don't cover natural therapies in many countries, we're obliged to pay out of our own pockets, to attend a natural clinic. However good health doesn't have to be expensive and is our best weapon when it comes to cancer prevention. A good diet, low in sugar and high in vegetables and fruits is the basis for health. Exercise to stimulate the lymphatic system and strengthen the heart, lungs and muscles is also high on the list. Supplements of vitamins, minerals and antioxidants will make up for any shortfalls in our diets, and for the lack of nutrition in our foods. Last, but certainly not least, probiotics and enzymes will help us digest these nutrients for maximum availability, and strip cancer stem cells of their protective protein coating so that the immune system can seek and destroy them.

There is more - much more. There is not enough space in one chapter to do justice to this subject.

I have provided a list of natural doctors below. Do your own research and draw your own conclusions. Being informed will help you from making a hasty decision.

Sources:

http://www.vitalitylink.com/article-chelation-therapy-2080-intravenous-vitamin-cancer-cells-dose-high

The Enzyme Treatment of Cancer and its Scientific Basis. Dr. John Beard

https://draxe.com/probiotic-foods/

http://www.coreonehealth.com/chronic-digestive-system-disorders

https://thetruthaboutcancer.com/the-cancer-oxygen-connectionoxygen-to-kill-cancer/

https://www.cancertutor.com/ozone/

http://articles.mercola.com/sites/articles/archive/2011/08/21/enzymes-special-report.aspx

Dr. N Gonzales M.D.

Chapter 8 – Alzheimer's

"The intuitive mind is a sacred gift, and the rational mind its faithful servant. We have created a society that honors the servant and has forgotten the gift" - Albert Einstein

A survey has found older people are more afraid of dementia, specifically Alzheimer's, than any other disease. Fear of heart disease and cancer come further down the list, even though they claim more lives each year than Alzheimer's.

Alzheimer's is a big scary, little-understood condition, where people lose their sense of reality. They don't recognize their loved ones and live in a shadowy, twilight world that most of us cannot even begin to comprehend. It gets worse over time and is eventually fatal. So, let's shine a light on Alzheimer's and dementia, so we can better understand it, and remove some of the mystery and fear.

Alzheimer's is one form of dementia, which is an umbrella term that describes a set of mental and neurocognitive conditions. Dementia and Alzheimer's are often used interchangeably, and I have used both terms in this chapter. The good news is Alzheimer's is *not a natural part of aging*, and there is a lot we can do to prevent and manage this disease.

Have you ever walked into a room, then been unable to remember what you were doing there? This is perfectly normal, and not a sign of dementia. The same can be said for losing your car keys, forgetting to feed the cat (or the kids!) These little lapses in memory are usually caused by having too much on our minds and are nothing to worry about.

If you're having difficulty performing familiar tasks, feeling confused about time, or are having speech problems, then it might be a good idea to chat with your doctor. *Don't make yourself miserable worrying about it;* there is a lot that can be done, and it's far better to be diagnosed in the early stages. There is a simple test that you can take, called the clock drawing test, here -

https://www.verywell.com/the-clock-drawing-test-98619

What is Alzheimer's?

Alzheimer's is thought to be caused by a buildup of *beta-amyloid plaque* or *protein fibrils* in the brain. These are sticky substances which block the normal communication between nerve synapses and cause the eventual death of brain cells.

What are the risk factors?

- Having a family history of the disease

- Brain injury

- Age

There is nothing we can do to alter the above, but there are other risk factors which are under our control (modifiable).

- Smoking

- Elevated cholesterol

- High blood pressure (hypertension)

- Heart disease

- Lack of exercise

- Obesity

How to prevent and manage Alzheimer's Disease

While there are medications that treat Alzheimer's (cholinesterase inhibitors), it's better to prevent this disease. There are many natural ways to prevent Alzheimer's, and they are listed here.

DHA - This is an Omega-3 fatty acid which makes up a large part of the fats in the human brain. Evidence suggests DHA can help prevent Alzheimer's by reducing beta-amyloid plaques from forming. DHA is an important structural component of the brain, particularly the *cerebral cortex*. The cerebral cortex is responsible for memory, creativity, emotion, and judgment, among other functions. DHA is found in oily fish such as salmon, tuna, trout, mackerel, and sardines. You can also supplement with fish or Krill oil. Low DHA levels have been linked to memory loss, Alzheimer's, schizophrenia depression and bipolar disorder.

While the brain requires both Omega-3 and Omega-6 fats, our typical diet is usually much higher is Omega-6; the average being 1:25. Omega-6 is found in vegetable oils, such as canola and safflower. This imbalance can cause inflammation in the body, including the brain. The ideal ratio is 1:1 omega 3/6. Cutting out vegetable oils and taking fish or Krill oils should go a long way to help restore this balance.

Resveratrol – Resveratrol is made from red wine extracts and is perhaps the best supplement we can take at this time, to prevent Alzheimer's. Resveratrol produces *sirtuins* which mimic the beneficial effect of *calorific reduction* (lowering calorie intake). In 2015 *Neurology* published a large nationwide clinical trial on patients taking high doses of resveratrol. It was found that long-term resveratrol treatment appeared to stop, or at least slow, the progress of patients with mild to moderate Alzheimer's. Alzheimer's sufferers have brains that are inflamed. This could be partly due to the immune system response to the plaque build-up. Resveratrol contains polyphenols, which reduce inflammation.

While the slow wheels of scientific research continue to turn on Resveratrol, there is absolutely no need to wait before taking it. It is perfectly safe to take in the recommended dose, and can only enhance your health. However, it's not a cheap supplement.

Coconut oil – All our organs need fat, our brain especially. Human brains are composed of sixty percent fat by weight. Some experts believe low-fat diets may be responsible for the increase in brain disorders such as anxiety, depression, and Alzheimer's. To remain in peak condition, the cell membranes need healthy fats; an example being medium chain triglycerides (MCTs). Furthermore, our brains can't store energy, so they need a constant supply. Even though the brain is a small part of the human body, it uses twenty percent of our daily energy output. This is where coconut oil is so useful.

Coconut oil is a rich source of medium chain triglycerides. These are then broken down by the liver to produce ketones, which are a great source of brain energy. Although the brain uses glucose as a primary source of energy, as we age our brains become less able to process glucose as brain fuel. Ketones can produce the energy the brain needs to function, as they readily cross the blood-brain barrier.

Alzheimer's patients have brain inflammation which further slows their brain's ability to process glucose as fuel as the cells have become insulin resistant. This is often referred to as *type 3 diabetes*. This resistance leads to cell die-off and further damage to the brain. When ketones are used as an alternative source of energy to glucose, it bypasses the need for insulin. Pet scans have proven that areas of the brain affected by Alzheimer's, rapidly takes up ketones as an energy source.

One way to produce ketones is to adopt a diet that contains proteins and fats, with little to no carbohydrates; known as a *ketogenic diet,* or *keto* for short. However, few people want to go on such an extreme diet for any length of time. Coconut oil and its medium chain triglycerides provide another way to get MCTs into the body.

Scientists at the Byrd Alzheimer's Institute at the University of South Florida are investigating the effect coconut oil has on the brain, and if it can provide some clues to curing Alzheimer's and other forms of dementia. Coconut oil has previously had a bad name due to scientific studies carried out in the mid-1990s. However, these studies used *hydrogenated* coconut oil, not the virgin variety available today. Hydrogenated coconut oil has been refined for storage purposes and has a different in molecular structure. *Never buy hydrogenated coconut oil.* It has the same nasty side effects as hydrogenated vegetable oil, such as clogged arteries and inflammation. Populations that traditionally use virgin coconut oil as a base for cooking are exceptionally healthy, with low incidences of diseases like dementia, cancer, heart disease and diabetes.

For a real-life story on how a doctor kept her husband's dementia at bay with coconut oil, follow this link –

https://www.ihealthtube.com/video/dr-mary-newport-coconut-oil-alzheimers-treatment

Foods that help prevent Alzheimer's

Leafy greens – Spinach, collard and other greens are high in folate (folic acid), which has found to be at low levels in dementia patients. Folate lowers *homocysteine* levels in the blood, which triggers inflammation, thought to increase risk of dementia and heart disease.

Cruciferous vegetables - Broccoli, Brussel sprouts, kale, cauliflower, and bok-choy. These have a wealth of vitamins, minerals, and folate. Folate is one of the many B vitamins in the group called vitamin B complex. A deficiency in folate is associated with depression and dementia, and low levels of folate can lead to faster deterioration in cognitive brain function. For best effect, folate should be combined with vitamin B12.

Beans and legumes – Lentils, kidney beans, split peas, mung beans etc. High in protein, these also contain choline, a B vitamin that boosts *acetylcholine*, which is a neurotransmitter critical for brain function. Beans and legumes contain folate, iron, magnesium, and potassium.

Whole grains – All whole grains are beneficial. Gluten free options are kammut, quinoa, and oats. Stay clear of processed cereals which are made from simple, or processed carbohydrates.

Cherries - These berries contain *anthocyanin* that protects the brain from damage caused by free radicals. They have anti-inflammatory properties and contain antioxidants, vitamin C and vitamin E. Other berries are also recommended.

Brightly colored vegetables - Pumpkin, tomatoes, squash, beetroot and carrots. These vegetables contain vitamin A, folate, and iron, that help with cognition. Steam, or stir fry until just cooked.

Nuts – Pecans, almonds, walnuts, cashews, and hazelnuts. All contain omega 3 and omega 6, vitamin E, vitamin B6, folate and magnesium. Nuts need to be kept fresh in the fridge.

Seeds – Pumpkin and sunflower seeds. These contain vitamin E, zinc, and choline.

Spices – Turmeric, cinnamon, cumin, and sage. These can all help to break up brain plaque and reduce brain inflammation too. Some can be taken as capsules which are a more concentrated form.

Protein – Protein foods, whether animal or plant based, contain amino acids. These are used by the brain to produce neurotransmitters, which enable the network of cells in the brain to communicate. Protein also builds the hormones and enzymes that control all the body's processes. For those who don't eat animal flesh, whey protein powder makes a nice shake, with some berries thrown in. Vegans can use soy or pea protein powders.

Foods to avoid

Smoked or processed meats, such as ham and bacon contain *nitrosamines*. High levels of nitrosamines have been linked to diseases such as dementia, Parkinson's, and diabetes.

Foods made from white flour – bread, pasta, baked goods etc.

Beer - Beer contains nitrites, which can increase the risk of Alzheimer's.

Margarine – Use butter or olive oil instead.

Sugar - Yes, our 'sweet' old friend has been linked to dementia. Without getting too scientific, a protective enzyme in the brain is damaged by a process called *glycation*. Simply put, high glucose levels in the brain leaves us more vulnerable to Alzheimer's.

Exercise

There's no getting away from it. Exercise is simply good for everything! Many studies have suggested improved brain function and slowing of dementia symptoms in people who exercise.

There's no need to slog away at the gym if gym's not your thing. Simple walking for 20-30 minutes a day will do it. Combine this with some upper body stretching to make sure all the muscles are involved. Yoga, Pilates, or swimming are gentle exercises which exercise the whole body. If you haven't exercised in a while, start slowly, and work up. Exercise is also a great stress reliever. Stress puts an extra load on our bodies, including our brain.

Research into Alzheimer's is ongoing, albeit slowly. Reduce the risk and the worry, by employing the advice in this chapter.

Sources:

https://www.ncbi.nlm.nih.gov/pmc/articles/PMC1123448/

http://www.umm.edu/health/medical/altmed/supplement/vitamin-b9-folic-acid

https://www.ncbi.nlm.nih.gov/books/NBK22436/

https://bebrainfit.com/coconut-oil-dementia/

http://www.news.com.au/lifestyle/health/health-problems/excess-sugar-linked-to-alzheimers-study-finds-a-tipping-point/news-story/365c27ebdc3d2f251dda260e2f3122a9

https://www.fightdementia.org.au/about-dementia/health-professionals/the-essentials

https://en.wikipedia.org/wiki/Docosahexaenoic_acid

https://www.sciencedaily.com/releases/2016/07/160718133005.htm

https://draxe.com/kamut/

http://www.dailymail.co.uk/health/article-3352079/Pill-wash-away-cause-Alzheimer-s-Treatment-dissolves-toxic-plaques-brain-warning-sign-disease.html

http://www.alzheimers.net/2014-01-02/foods-that-induce-memory-loss/

http://www.webmd.com/alzheimers/news/20020301/folic-acid-may-help-prevent-alzheimers

Heneka MT, Carson MJ, El Khoury J, et al. Neuroinflammation in Alzheimer's Disease. The Lancet 2015;14:388-405.

http://www.medscape.com/viewarticle/851172

http://www.ncbi.nlm.nih.gov/pmc/articles/PMC4005962/

https://www.sciencedaily.com/releases/2009/07/090705215239.htm

https://bebrainfit.com/mct-oil-benefits-brain/

Chapter 9 - Heart Disease

"A good heart is better than all the heads in the world" - Edward G. Bulwer-Lytton

Even though heart disease is one of the biggest lifestyle diseases of modern times, people tend to fear this less than cancer or Alzheimer's disease. Maybe it's because there's less mystery concerned with heart disease, however it's just as deadly. The good news is, heart disease (apart from congenital heart disease) is preventable, and that's what we're going to look at here.

Heart disease or cardiovascular disease is a broad term that includes multiple diseases affecting the heart.

- coronary heart disease

- heart attack

- heart failure

- stroke

- arrhythmias – abnormal heart beats

- aneurysm – a bulge caused by weakening of the heart muscle or artery

- septal defect – an abnormal opening between the left and right sides of the heart

- peripheral vascular disease – a disease of the large blood vessels of the arms, legs, and feet

Preventing all kinds of heart disease depends on our daily lifestyle habits. These boil down to what we eat and how much we move. A healthy diet will keep our blood sugar and blood pressure low and keep down triglyceride levels, which can block arteries. There are risk factors that are outside our control, such as age and inherited heart defects, but many are within our control by substituting unhealthy habits with better ones. (See the chapter on diet, which goes more thoroughly into developing healthy eating habits).

Risk factors that we *can* control -

Smoking

"Did you know that in the U.S. alone, tobacco kills the equivalent of three jumbo jets full of people crashing every day, with no survivors."
– Pritiken.com

Scary, isn't it? Smoking doubles the risk of heart disease. Just cutting out this habit can dramatically reduce your risk. It doesn't matter how old you are, or how long, or even how many cigarettes, you've smoked. It's *never too late* to give up tobacco. The body's healing powers are amazing and our hearts can begin to repair mere hours after stopping.

Why does smoking affect your heart? Tobacco smoke contains a host of toxic substances, including carbon monoxide, which reduces the amount of oxygen in the blood. The heart must therefore work harder to supply the body with the oxygen it needs. This puts the heart under stress. Tobacco smoke contains nicotine which stimulates adrenaline production. This also causes a raised heartbeat and may also cause high blood pressure. Smoking can damage the arterial lining, causing a build-up of plaque which narrows the arteries. Smoking damages other organs in the body too, such as the lungs, liver, and kidneys.

Last, but not least, tobacco smoke makes the blood more likely to clot, raising the risk of heart attack or stroke.

It's not easy to quit, but for your health and the health of those around you, it's worth the effort. I'm an ex-smoker so I understand how hard it can be. Find a quit-smoking buddy, try hypnosis, and have a look at the chapter on energy medicine, which has some free resources on quitting.

High Blood Pressure

High blood pressure can be prevented without the use of drugs. If it's seriously high, seek the advice of your doctor of course. Natural methods are - losing some weight, reducing alcohol and switching from red meat, to chicken and fish. Regular exercise will help, both with high blood pressure, and with weight loss. Smoking can raise blood pressure too, so do try to give that up. The ideal resting blood pressure target is below 120/80.

There are mixed theories about how salt affects our blood pressure. Medical science is coming around to the opinion that salt, is not a cause on its own. Salt is necessary to maintain fluid balance. Salt also causes us to feel thirsty, so excess is flushed out through the kidneys. What is more important, is the balance between sodium (salt) and potassium. The ideal ratio is 1-part sodium to 2-parts potassium. Cutting out processed food and sodas and adding more fresh foods to your diet will help tremendously. High sources of potassium include all kinds of potatoes, watermelon, bananas, spinach, beets and even tomato sauce.

Magnesium and calcium are also important minerals to keep blood pressure in check. Magnesium is particularly useful to prevent heart attacks, as it helps relax artery walls. Calcium helps to regulate sodium levels in the blood.

The following foods, herbs and spices can help keep blood pressure low:

- Basil
- Cinnamon
- Cardamom
- Flaxseed
- Garlic
- Ginger

- Hawthorn

- Celery seed

- Turmeric

- Hibiscus (as a tea)

- Coconut Water

- Fish Oil

- Hawthorn

- Nuts

- Vitamin D

- Coenzyme Q10

- Acetyl-L-carnitine

Cholesterol

Cholesterol is a waxy substance found in all the cells of your body and in animal foods. Cholesterol is necessary to life, which is why the body makes the required amount it needs. Cholesterol travels through the bloodstream in packages known as lipoproteins. There are 2 types of lipoproteins, high-density lipoprotein, or HDL and low-density lipoprotein, or LDL. These are sometimes labeled as "good" and "bad" cholesterol, respectively.

Cholesterol is also found in certain animal-based foods, but this has very little impact on cholesterol levels in the blood.

If a doctor is concerned about a patient's high cholesterol levels, chances are the balance of LDL to HDL is high. This is said to increase the risk of heart attack. The LDL can clog artery walls (atherosclerosis) increasing the risk of heart attack and stroke, but this is mainly when the LDL becomes oxidized by the presence of free radicals.

Most people's cholesterol levels can be kept in a normal range by diet alone. In some cases, there is a family history of high cholesterol - *familial hypercholesterolaemia*, which may need to be lowered artificially, if it reaches extra high levels.

Magnesium is a mineral which can lower cholesterol levels, and has often been referred to as the "natural statin." As many people are lacking in this mineral, it may be a good idea to take magnesium supplements. Food sources of magnesium include brown rice, green leafy vegetables, green peas, nuts and seeds, beans, and soy.

Most doctors will insist that a diet high in saturated fat will increase cholesterol levels, but in fact it is sugar that's the real culprit, as it increases inflammation, leading to the oxidation of LDL.

In conclusion, the best way to keep cholesterol levels healthy and in balance is to cut out sugar, eat healthy, take a magnesium supplement and exercise. This is based on my own research only, so please be discerning, and be sure to look at both sides of the argument. The following articles make interesting reading.

http://www.zoeharcombe.com/the-knowledge/we-have-got-cholesterol-completely-wrong/

http://www.docsopinion.com/health-and-nutrition/lipids/ldl-c/

http://www.zoeharcombe.com/2016/11/familial-hypercholesterolemia-fh/

Blood sugar

Keeping blood sugar low, is crucial to heart health and for preventing type 2 diabetes and inflammation; both which have a serious negative effect on the heart. If your blood sugar levels are in the healthy range, you can keep them that way by exercising and cutting down on simple carbohydrates, such as white bread, white rice, and sugar. If it's on the high side, or if you have pre-diabetes, or diabetes type 2, cut out simple carbohydrates completely. Carbohydrates convert to sugar during the digestion process. This is one of the best and fastest ways to reducing blood sugar (glucose) levels.

Drink plenty of water during the day and keep your fiber intake high. Vegetables are high in fiber and should form a major part of your diet. Get creative with vegetables! Find some delicious vegetable recipes on-line, to add interest to your meals.

Fiber is indigestible and helps the passage of food through the intestines. It also helps quell the appetite without adding extra calories. There are two types of fiber, soluble and insoluble. The main difference is that soluble fiber dissolves in water. Soluble fiber is more capable of lowering blood glucose levels. Always drink plenty of water when consuming foods high in fiber.

What about complex carbohydrates?

These are "whole" grains, which have not been refined in any way. These are a valuable part of a healthy diet as they take much longer to break down. Some examples are oatmeal, barley, whole wheat, millet, buckwheat, kamut, quinoa and brown rice. Whole grains are a good source of fiber and B vitamins. Even diabetics can eat whole grains in moderation. I can just hear the anti-grain people growling here, but I'm simply stating the research.

Two important minerals that will help lower blood glucose are chromium and magnesium. Cinnamon is a spice which also helps keep glucose levels low.

Exercise

Exercise is vital for keeping our hearts healthy and strong. It's possible learn to enjoy exercise if you start with just a little every day – just trust me on this! Find an exercise you enjoy and find a suitable time to do it each day. Simple walking is great to get started, and some folks do nothing else. Walking is easy to slot into your day; walk to the next bus stop, walk up the stairs instead of using the lift. As soon as this becomes a habit, you'll do it without thinking.

Exercise is also a great way of lowering stress levels which can increase heart attack risk. Check the chapter on exercise for the different types of exercise and more suggestions.

This concludes our chapter on heart disease. I hope there's been something in here that will help you on your way to a healthier heart!

Sources:

https://www.pritikin.com/improving-heart-health-naturally

https://authoritynutrition.com/different-types-of-fiber/

http://www.docsopinion.com/health-and-nutrition/lipids/ldl-c/

http://www.dailyherald.com/article/20150207/entlife/150209666/

https://www.ncbi.nlm.nih.gov/pubmed/2194788

http://www.onegreenplanet.org/natural-health/a-guide-to-consuming-grains-for-diabetics-and-people-with-blood-sugar-issues/

http://www.naturalnews.com/022490_grains_sugar_blood.html

Chapter 10 - Chronic Pain

"One small crack doesn't mean that you are broken. It means that you were put to the test, and you didn't fall apart" – Linda Poindexter

One area of aging which particularly interests me is chronic pain. Mainly because I was a victim of it for over seven years. It's only recently I've managed to put this behind me, mainly by improving my posture. I don't treat clients for chronic pain myself, so I've invited someone who's been treating clients for many years and knows everything there is to know about human anatomy.

Interview with Kathryn Merrow – The Pain Relief Coach

"I'd like to welcome Kathryn Merrow, the Pain Relief Coach. Kathryn, could you tell us a bit about how you became interested in physical therapy? What started you on this journey?

Hi Wendy, I'm so glad to be with you today! I'm not actually interested in physical therapy. I do specialize in manual therapy. I work with muscles, helping them get back to being happy and healthy. Primarily, I do this by looking for the physical causes of someone's pain and getting rid of those causes.

We seem to have an epidemic of chronic pain, particularly back pain, these days. Ruling out injury, do you think there's anything we can do to prevent this? Is it our lifestyles that are causing all these aches and pains? Do we need to move around more?

Oh, Wendy, if you watch little children move you will know the answer! In fact, I know that YOU already do know the answer. Little children move all the time! It's hard to get most of them to slow down and stop moving. They use ALL the muscles. They climb. They run. They hop, jump, wiggle, and move almost every waking hour! But then we grow up. We go to school. We get a job. We stop moving and start sitting or standing for long hours. We get into pain because we get out of muscular balance. Most pain is caused by overuse, abuse, or underuse of muscles. Be a child!

There's been a lot of talk lately about sitting, and how dangerous it is. A lot of people really don't have much choice though. They sit in their car to get to work, they sit all day at a desk, then back in their car again. They're so tired in the evening, all they feel like doing is sitting in front of the TV. What advice can you give people whose jobs almost force them to be sedentary?

It's called The Sitting Disease. *Dis-Ease*. Your body is no longer at ease. It happens when we get stuck in those sitting positions. I love telling the story of my friend, Rosalie. She had the sitting disease. She did just what you said, sat all day, sat at work, in the car, at dinner, and when she watched television. She had pain in her hips and many health challenges. How did she get better? She started walking. And at first, all she could do was walk in her home. Eventually, she walked around her yard. Soon she was able to walk a bit down the street and back. The distance and her speed continued to expand, and she continued to feel better and her health challenges became less. One of her doctors said, "Rosalie, no one who comes to see me ever gets better but you are getting better!" I talk about her more in my *Walking Smart* program. I love to share stories about people healing naturally. Bodies heal all the time! I am not saying that movement or massage or a healthy diet can cure everything. Unfortunately, a few things aren't fixable naturally, but most of our pain problems are caused by muscles and muscles ARE treatable!

Great answer, and I think this was 90% my own problem! I've actually invested in a standing desk for my computer, and I stop and walk around every 45 minutes. It's made a huge difference. One more question - What tips would you give an older adult who has never exercised much in her life, but now wants to start?

Start slowly! I have a colleague who used to be a competitive body builder. When she would talk with groups of chronic pain patients, she would tell them to start with one repetition. And someone would always say, "One? One repetition won't do anything!" And she would reply, "That's true. But tomorrow you won't be sore and you can do one more. And after a few days of doing just one, you can do two." A big problem with exercise programs is that people go overboard trying to get back in shape all at once. It doesn't happen. Do you know how many women I have seen who could hardly walk because they did the *Buns of Steel* program all the way through on the first try?

And there was the woman who came in with pain and couldn't figure it out because all she did was take a walk. I asked her how far she went. "Oh, 5 miles," she said, "But I always used to walk 5 miles." I asked how long it had been since she walked last. "Well, it had been several years." And that's why she hurt. So, start slowly. It's not a race. And move consistently. Did you know that when you are watching television or sitting at your desk you don't have to be still? Be like that little child. Wiggle your toes and fingers, spread them. Circle your hands, stretch your fingers. Lift your leg and twirl your foot in one direction and then in the other. Flex your calf muscles. Lift your toes. Squeeze your buttock muscles so that you bounce up and down a bit in your chair. Do that at traffic lights, too. You don't have to work hard to move your muscles. Some people get confused looks on their faces when they are trying to contract a specific muscle. They used to be able to do it and they can learn to do it again; it will just take a little practice.

When you sit so much, your posture tends to slump. That causes weak back muscles so one of my very favorite moves in the whole world is to sit with your breastbone lifted, shoulders relaxed, and squeeze your shoulder blades toward your spine. That movement strengthens your back muscles and we need strong backs. We need strong backs and strong legs. They support us. We have to support them so they can support us, throughout our whole life.

Kathryn, that's excellent advice. Now how do people find you? Do you have a website where you dispense all your wisdom? Can people book a session with you on your site? Otherwise, is there a phone number that they can contact you on?

My main website is http://www.kathrynmerrow.com/. That contain links to my other sites too. http://walkingsmart.com/ is my site, specifically on walking.

Thanks a lot for speaking with us today Katherine. You really do know your stuff! Kathrine's site contains a wealth of pain resources, and her newsletter also provides some especially useful tips on pain relief, together with a free report. The sign-up form is on the main page."

TENS therapy -

TENS is an effective, drug-free method for relieving pain. TENS equipment is used is many physiotherapy clinics, but hand-held devices can also be purchased for use at home. TENS is an abbreviation for *transcutaneous electrical nerve stimulation*, or stimulation of nerves through the skin. A tiny electrical current causes a mild tingling sensation, that emits from the TENS device, through wires to self-adhesive pads, which are placed near the source of the pain.

Other techniques for managing or curing chronic pain

- Reduce weight

- Improve posture

- Exercise regularly

- Eat a well-balanced diet

- Learn to manage stress

- Practice correct lifting techniques

Alternative healing systems for pain relief

It's so easy to take pain medication, but the side effects over the long term are not good. Alternative healing systems are a different approach to pain relief, that a lot of people have tried, and found success with. There are two types of alternative healing systems I recommend, and these are Eutaptics© and PSTEC. For more details and a how-to, see the chapter on alternative healing systems. But first check with your doctor to make sure the pain is not something more serious.

When using alternative healing systems for pain relief, it's best to address the emotions surrounding the pain, before addressing the pain directly, such as frustration, anger, disappointment, sadness, or grief. This will clear the stress that usually accompanies chronic pain, even when we're not consciously aware of it. Alternative healing systems even work for pain from accidents, fibromyalgia, cancer pain, in fact, any pain at all.

PSTEC also addresses pain relief and has a lot of success stories on the relief of pain. A real case study can be found here - https://www.youtube.com/watch?v=MPiBRF0wZEI

Our mind and body are connected. Our typical approach to chronic pain, has been to treat the body only. By looking at the emotional response to pain, many cures have been possible.

Sources:

http://pstecaudiosource.org/pstecstory-Sara.html (audio)

http://superchangeyourlife.com/interviews/interviews-tim-phizackerley/ (video)

http://undergroundhealthreporter.com/eft-therapy-tapping/

https://www.painmanagement.org.au/2014-09-11-13-35-53/2014-09-11-13-36-47/183-transcutaneous-electrical-nerve-stimulation-tens.html

https://www.mindbodygreen.com/0-18206/how-tapping-can-help-relieve-chronic-pain.html

https://my.clevelandclinic.org/health/articles/chronic-myofascial-pain-cmp

http://www.the-energy-healing-site.com/natural-pain-relief.html

Chapter 11 - Depression

"I wanted to talk about it. Damn it. I wanted to scream. I wanted to yell. I wanted to shout about it. But all I could was whisper, "I'm fine." – HealthyPlace.com

There is nothing worse than being depressed! We have all felt this from time to time, but to be stuck in a state of unhappiness continuously, is tragic. The world seems like a colorless place, and it can feel like your soul is being crushed. Being told to "snap out of it," seems cruel, and it is. People can't simply snap out of a depressed state.

However, there are many ways to help depression, and if depression is affecting you, I'd like to help.

There are many different types of depression. Events in our lives can cause unhappiness, and negative thoughts can make life look so bleak, some people feel suicidal. Life doesn't always go the way we want it to, and there are events that will make even the most positive people feel depressed; a death in the family, a child who takes drugs or the loss of a job. It's perfectly natural to feel upset at these times.

Then there is "clinical" or major depression. This can cause people to feel depressed, even when there's no apparent reason for it. There are various types of clinical depression including post-natal depression, bipolar disorder, seasonal affective disorder, or *SAD*, in which lack of light is believed to affect mood.

Clinical depression is what I want to discuss here, because there are ways to cure depression without taking "anti-depressants" such as *Prozac*, which can actually make some people feel worse. Prozac is just one of a class of drugs called *serotonin reuptake Inhibitors* (SSRIs), which aim to increase levels of serotonin in the brain. While these drugs work well for some people, it can cause agitation and other side effects in others. Some people even become suicidal while taking SSRIs. Remember, *no drug is without risk.*

Serotonin is a neurotransmitter that can maintain mood balance. It transmits impulses between nerve cells, creating moods of well-being and happiness. Too much serotonin can have the opposite effect, leading to high anxiety, seizures, and other side effects. This is known as *serotonin toxicity*, or *serotonin syndrome.* This is why it's better to obtain serotonin from the natural sources, listed below. Some of these contain tryptophan, which is an amino acid which converts to serotonin in the body.

Healthy fats – These includes Omega 3 oils from fish, or Krill. Coconut oil is another option.

Proteins – Include enough protein in your diet, particularly high tryptophan foods, such as turkey, chicken, red meat, cheese, eggs, and tofu.

Pineapple – This fruit contains tryptophan, as well as digestive enzymes.

Nuts and seeds – All types.

Grains - Oats, wheatgerm and buckwheat

Legumes – Beans and lentils

There are also herbs which can help with depression:

St. John's wort – 300 mg three times a day.

Hawthorn

Ginkgo biloba

California poppy

Lavender – use as an essential oil, not to be taken.

Purple passionflower

Chamomile – makes a relaxing tea

Lemon balm

What else can we do?

Avoid caffeine, which can reduce serotonin levels. L-Tyrosine is an amino acid which can boost your energy in the same way as caffeine. Switch to green tea which contains *L-Theanine*. L-Theanine has a relaxing and calming effect.

Unstable blood sugar can cause mood swings. If that's you, then make sure you don't go too long between meals.

Movement creates endorphins. A brisk walk can lift mood. In fact, *any* exercise will work.

Watch your thinking. Monitor your thoughts throughout the day. Are they all negative? See if you can make a list of positive thoughts you can concentrate on instead. It takes practice, but in a few weeks, you'll be feeling a lot better.

Natural treatments for depression

5-HTP – Start with 50 mg, up to 300 mg if necessary. 5-HTP converts directly into serotonin. Symptoms that are similar to serotonin toxicity can occur if you take too much. Don't take 5-HTP with any other anti-depressant drugs.

SAMe – start with 200mg on an empty stomach twice a day. Increase your dose slowly over two weeks to a maximum of 600mg twice a day. SAMe can be expensive, but also highly effective. Side effects over the recommended dose are similar to those experienced with 5-HTP.

Make sure your hormones are in balance. Hormone imbalance can directly affect your mood. There are simple tests your doctor can do for the thyroid, adrenal and sex hormones. The main hormones to test for are TSH, free T4, free T3, total T3, thyroid antibodies, cortisol, DHEA-S, pregnenolone, estradiol, progesterone, and testosterone. Yes, us women have testosterone, just in smaller amounts than men.

Speak to a trusted friend or a counselor about your concerns. Talking can be therapeutic, and may put your problems in a better perspective.

Acupuncture is based in traditional Chinese medicine and can work well for depression. Acupuncture is based on the theory that, in a depressed person, energy, or *Qi*, is disrupted along the meridians, or energy channels of the body. Fine needles are placed at various points of the body to normalize the Qi.

In some cases of serious depression, medication may be the only option. If that's the case, make sure your doctor checks out all aspects of your health, to ensure there's no other factor that may be contributing to your condition.

Depression is a complex condition. I hope that the above advice can bring you some peace of mind.

Sources:

http://www.berkeleywellness.com/supplements/other-supplements/article/theanine-calmness-pill

http://www.medicalnewstoday.com/kc/serotonin-facts-232248

http://www.webmd.com/depression/ssris-myths-and-facts-about-antidepressants#1

https://psychcentral.com/lib/acupuncture-anxiety-depression/

https://www.beyondblue.org.au/the-facts/depression/types-of-depression

https://www.psychologytoday.com/blog/owning-pink/201103/11-natural-treatments-depression-md-s-tips-skipping-the-prozac

http://www.healthline.com/health/healthy-sleep/foods-that-could-boost-your-serotonin#nuts7

http://www.webmd.com/depression/guide/depression-types#1

http://www.ncbi.nlm.nih.gov/pubmed/24051231

Errington-Evans, N. (2011). Acupuncture for anxiety. CNS Neuroscience and Therapeutics, 18(4), 277-284. doi: 10.1111/j.1755-5949.2011.00254.x

Chapter 12 - Osteoporosis

Weight-bearing exercise builds bone density, builds your muscular strength so that you can hold your body up where those bones have a tendency to get weak." Ann Richards

Osteoporosis literally means "porous bone." It's a condition where the body either loses bone tissue or fails to replace it. Osteoporotic bones have lost their density and are weak and more likely to break or fracture. Osteoporosis is a silent disease, and sometimes the first we know about it is when we break a bone after a fall, and the doctor tells you it's due to osteoporosis. This is why it's important for those of us over fifty, to ask for a bone mineral density test (BMD), particularly if we don't exercise, don't eat dairy produce, or don't get much sun exposure.

The most common areas affected by bone fractures are the wrist, spine, and hips.

Bones are dynamic, living tissue and are in a content state of growth and change. Bones consist mainly of collagen, together with calcium phosphate and carbonate. Inside the bone is the marrow, which is where red and white blood cells and platelets are manufactured.

A less severe form of osteoporosis is called *osteopenia*. Osteopenia is simply less drastic form of osteoporosis and may develop into osteoporosis if steps aren't taken to prevent this.

Certain health conditions can predispose us to developing both these diseases. A few of these are celiac disease, rheumatoid arthritis, multiple sclerosis, breast or prostate cancer and diabetes. There are medications that may also place us under increased risk. These include, methotrexate, antacids that contain aluminum, selective serotonin reuptake inhibitors (SSRIs) for depression and steroids for arthritis. This is by no means a full list.

What causes osteopenia and osteoporosis?

- Age

- Long-term use of certain medications

- Smoking

- Hormonal imbalances

- Low vitamin D levels

- Low calcium levels

- Emotional stress

- Dietary deficiencies

- Chemotherapy

Natural remedies for osteoporosis

There is no cure for osteoporosis, but it can be slowed, and the degeneration of bone tissue can be stopped. It's easy to feel that it's too late to do anything after a diagnosis, but there's plenty we can do, so read on.

Bones need to be used to grow strong. Like muscles, bones strengthen according to the demands we place on them. Bones respond especially well to weight training. This could be lifting weights, or using bodyweight exercises. However, any exercise that forces the bones to work against gravity are also useful; walking, climbing stairs, dancing and hiking are some examples. Swimming, while a great exercise for health, doesn't contribute a great deal towards increasing bone mass, as there is no load on the bones themselves. However, swimming can be combined with weight training three times a week for at least thirty minutes. If you own a vibration platform, this has been shown to increase bone mass too, and is a good idea for those who can't do traditional exercise for any reason.

If you've been diagnosed with osteoporosis, it's important to prevent falls as much as you possibly can. Have support bars in the shower stall, and watch the floor for anything that may cause you to trip and fall.

Manage your stress levels. We all experience some stress, but when stress is constant, it's known as chronic. Chronic stress releases a stress hormone known as cortisol which can depress the bone-building osteoblasts, thus less new bone tissue is formed. Chronic stress affects our general health in many negative ways. Read the chapter on stress for some idea on how to alleviate chronic stress.

Heavy metals can replace bone minerals

Our body need certain metals in small amounts to thrive. Iron, zinc and copper are essential in the body as they maintain normal physiological functions. Other metals, though, are toxic to the body, such as lead, manganese, mercury, and cadmium; these are known as primary neurotoxins. These metals are absorbed into the body through smoking, pesticides and polluted air, food, or water. Mercury can be found in fish and even in dental amalgam fillings. Cadmium is found in car exhaust fumes and cigarette smoke. Lead has now been removed from gasoline in many countries, but remains in the soil, from where it contaminates any food grown in contaminated areas.

Toxic metals can take over mineral receptors in the bones, thus decreasing the levels of these essential bone-building minerals. Heavy metals can be detected in the body by analyzing hair or fingernail clippings.

Radium is another toxic metal than can lodge in bone tissue

Chelation is the fastest process which can help remove heavy metals from the body, and may be necessary if there's a heavy build up. Other options are:

Chlorella is a type of green algae which can also remove toxic metals when taken orally in sufficient doses.

Modified citrus pectin (MCP) will also help absorb heavy metals and remove them from the body. *Methylsulfonylmetahne*, or MSM, also works well as a detoxifier. These methods will take longer than chelation, but can also be used every few months to maintain a heavy-metal free system.

Whichever method you choose be sure to drink a lot of water to help flush out the toxic metals and protect the kidneys. Exercising for twenty minutes daily will also help to flush out toxins.

Foods that nourish our bones

The first step towards having strong bones is to eat a balanced diet. Include all the food groups, protein, carbohydrates and healthy fats. There's a lot of information about these food groups in the chapter on diet. Cut out processed foods as much as possible as they're high in salt and can upset the sodium/potassium balance.

As much of our bone tissue is made from calcium, foods containing calcium should take precedence if we're strengthening our bones. Apart from dairy foods, good sources of calcium are leafy green vegetables, legumes, canned salmon, nuts and seeds, oranges, and whole grains. Incorporate plenty of these into your diet, if you are lactose intolerant, or prefer not to eat dairy foods. There is a theory that milk is a bad choice for obtaining calcium, due to its acidifying effect on the body. Proponents of the acid/alkaline theory believe that certain foods, for example dairy and red meat, have an acidifying effect on the blood, and create a condition called *low-grade metabolic acidosis*. They also claim that disease cannot exist on a PH balanced environment.

I'm not one hundred percent sure about this, but include it here so you can make your own decisions. If the body is too acid, alkalizing minerals, like calcium, will be released from the bones' osteoclasts, in an attempt to neutralize the PH balance.

A list of acid foods can be seen here:

https://www.healthline.com/health/acid-foods-to-avoid

If you want to hedge your bets, like I do, simply eating plenty of alkaline foods should offset the acid effects of dairy foods. Alkaline foods include most vegetables, some fruits, apple cider vinegar, and sprouts. Some of these foods, for example lemons, may have an acid taste, but have an alkalizing effect in the body.

What supplements should we take to prevent bone loss?

Taking supplements to strengthen bones adds a safety net if your diet is low in the above foods. We tend to absorb less nutrients from food as we age. Add to this, the lack of nutrients in the soils due to over-farming, and it's likely that you may be lacking in some areas.

Some herbal remedies can interact with drugs, so always consult your doctor if you are taking any medication.

Calcium

There is no doubt that calcium is one of the most important minerals when it comes to bone strength, but taking calcium supplements has come into question lately, due to its tendency to circulate in the arteries, creating blockages, or *calcification*. Combining calcium with vitamins K2 and magnesium, will ensure calcium is absorbed by the bone tissues, where it can best be put to use.

Calcium is also beneficial for maintaining healthy blood vessels and regulating both blood pressure and blood glucose levels. Calcium comes in a range of different forms, with some being more available than others. Calcium *carbonate* is poorly absorbed, unless taken with food, whereas calcium *citrate* is well absorbed by the body. Aim for around 1,000 milligrams daily.

Vitamin D3

Vitamin D3 is essential for the absorption of calcium. This vitamin can be produced in the body by the action of sunlight on the skin. For those who spend most days indoors, or those with darker skins, supplements of D3 are essential. The same applies for countries that don't have much daylight in the winter months. Vitamin D3 is the natural form of the vitamin and is oil soluble, so 5,000 IU a day should be more than enough.

Vitamin K2

Vitamin K2 is essential for calcium and vitamin D3 for effectively use in the body. Vitamin K2 acts in synergy with calcium and vitamin D3 to prevent bone fractures. It directs calcium into the bones, rather than circulating in the coronary arteries, where it can form arterial plaque. Vitamin K2 is not stored in the body but is available through most green vegetables and a small amount in olive oil. Deficiency is rare in those consuming a healthy diet but can exist in those taking anticoagulant drugs. If supplementing, aim for 80 micrograms daily.

Boron

Boron is a mineral that the body uses as an 'activator'. Boron helps as a cofactor to convert vitamin D into its active form and increases absorption of calcium. In people with osteoporosis, boron can help immensely in replacing lost calcium back into the bones. Plant based foods can provide boron, as long as the soil contains enough of this mineral. Bananas, kale, and lentils are some examples of foods high in boron. Boron can be toxic in high amounts, so take care with supplements, as there is no advised dosage. Boron is best taken together with calcium and magnesium, but it's best to stick to food sources.

Magnesium

Magnesium is necessary for keeping the bones strong, and for absorption and metabolism of calcium. Sixty percent of our magnesium is stored in the bones and is released into the blood stream when levels fall below a certain level. Taking calcium supplements is much safer when your magnesium levels are high. It's best to take these minerals together, so that they can interact with each other. Magnesium acts in a similar way as boron, converting vitamin D into its active form. Even a slight magnesium deficiency can significantly accelerate the risk of osteoporosis. Magnesium performs many functions in the body, and surveys have indicated that up to eighty percent of the US population could be magnesium deficient.

Magnesium is found in leafy green vegetables, yogurt, black beans, almonds, avocados, and bananas. If supplementing, aim for 500 mg. Magnesium is considered one of the safer minerals to supplement.

Strontium

Strontium both thickens and strengthens bones. Thicker bones are not necessarily an advantage, as they could lose their tensile strength. Be careful of supplements that contain strontium, as this mineral does have some unpleasant side effects, and it may interfere with calcium absorption. Less is more, in the case of strontium. Therefore, food sources are safer than supplements. Strontium is found in seafood and root vegetables.

Horsetail

Horsetail is a herb that contains silicon and is often prescribed by natural doctors to stimulate bone regeneration.

Soy Isoflavones

Soy isoflavones can be found in soy milk and tofu. Research tends to support the beneficial effects of soy isoflavones on osteoporosis and this is probably due to its estrogenic effect. People at risk of breast cancer should avoid soy isoflavones. Soy can also cause allergic reactions in some individuals, although fermented soy is less likely to cause these reactions.

Prescription medications for osteoporosis

Some of the most common drugs prescribed for osteoporosis include, Alendronate (Fosamax), Ibandronate (Boniva), Zoledronic acid (Reclast) and Risedronate (Actonel). These come under the banner of phosphorous based, *bisphosphonates*. The purpose of these is to slow the action of *osteoclasts*, whose natural function is the breakdown of bone tissue, and allow the *osteoblasts*, that build new bone tissue, to 'catch up', thus building stronger bones.

While this sounds great in theory, the reality may be somewhat different. Our bones were designed to rebuild themselves constantly, by replacing old, worn out bone tissue with healthy new tissue. When the old bone cells are not discarded, the new tissue is laid down on a weak foundation. This produces bones that may appear denser, but they become thicker and more brittle. This increases the risk of fractures, specifically of the femur (thigh bone) – the very thing these drugs are supposed to prevent.

At the same time, osteoporosis drugs come with a library of side effects.

One of the worst of these side effects is *osteonecrosis of the jaw* (ONJ). Symptoms include jaw pain, infection and abscesses, as the jawbone is exposed inside the mouth. This is not a common side effect, but one I would be unlikely to line up for!

Cancer of the esophagus is another serious side effect that may occur from taking bisphosphate drugs. The esophagus is part of the digestive tube between the throat and the stomach. Esophageal cancer usually remains undetected until its latter stages, making it harder to treat.

Rapid, irregular heartbeat is also associated with bisphosphonate use. A recent study has shown that use of bisphosphonates increased the risk of serious atrial fibrillation by forty percent.

Other side effects are joint and muscle pain, flatulence, stomach upsets and reflux. The answer to the latter, according to the manufacturers, is to drink a large glass of water, and remain upright thirty minutes to one hour, before eating some food to settle the stomach. It really makes you wonder why the body is trying so hard to rid itself of this medication!

It really is worth taking the natural path to bone health. Both osteopenia and osteoporosis can be prevented or stopped with good nutrition, mineral supplements, and exercise. The alternative is to take risky drugs. Drugs do have their place in medicine, but osteoporosis drugs are not worth the misery.

Sources:

https://www.britannica.com/science/bone-formation

https://saveourbones.com/top-5-reasons-why-you-should-never-take-osteoporosis-drugs/

https://draxe.com/alkaline-diet/

https://saveourbones.com/strontium-demistyfied/

http://articles.mercola.com/sites/articles/archive/2012/05/16/vitamins-d-and-k2-reduce-osteoporosis.aspx

http://cheflynda.com/2015/03/the-inexpensive-arthritis-osteoporosis-cure/

https://www.betterbones.com/bone-nutrition/magnesium/

https://www.betterbones.com/bone-nutrition/boron/

http://www.webmd.com/osteoporosis/guide/osteopenia-early-signs-of-bone-loss#1

http://www.naturalmedicinejournal.com/journal/2010-11/naturopathic-approaches-preventing-and-treating-osteoporosis

https://greatist.com/health/18-surprising-dairy-free-sources-calcium

https://www.ncbi.nlm.nih.gov/pmc/articles/PMC5153379/

http://www.healthline.com/health/osteoporosis-alternative-treatments

https://en.wikipedia.org/wiki/Metal_toxicity

http://www.healthknot.com/heavy_metals.html

http://www.breathing.com/articles/toxicmetals.htm

http://www.dreliaz.org/recommended-product/for-chelation-and-detoxification/

https://draxe.com/osteoporosis-diet-5-natural-treatments/

https://www.nof.org/patients/what-is-osteoporosis/

Sharma, Abhishek, M.D., et al. "Risk of Serious Atrial Fibrillation and Stroke With Use of Bisphosphonates".

Chapter 13 - Menopause

"Therapy helps, but screaming obscenities is faster and cheaper" –
Katie Horner.

Some people breeze through menopause without even noticing it; others
seem to have every unpleasant symptom under the sun.

I was in the latter group. It was 2006 when I first noticed the symptoms.
I was grumpy, I couldn't sleep, couldn't concentrate, I had hot flashes
and, to put it mildly, I was a wreck. I even asked my doctor for a
prescription for hormone replacement therapy (HRT). He, being a wise
person, offered no comment, but merely raised his eyebrows and started
typing on his keyboard.

I took the prescription and started feeling slightly better. I knew there
were probably better options, and that hormone replacement therapy
was never a long-term solution, but I didn't want to think about it. My
hot flashes were becoming less frequent and I was sleeping better. My
husband wasn't afraid of me anymore.

Eventually, I started writing again and life was returning to some
semblance of normality. It was also at a time when concerns were being
raised about the safety of hormone replacement therapy. I turned to my
library of natural treatments to try and find a natural solution, that had
some chance of working.

I tried a lot of things; some worked better than others. I eventually found
that combining a few things together worked best for me. Did I totally
get rid of all my symptoms? No. However, I did get to a place where I
was functioning normally, with only a few hot flashes to deal with.

Menopause is a process that we women all have to go through eventually. it's not a disease, it's a natural stage of a woman's life. Taking hormone replacement therapy (HRT), only delays the onset, and when you stop the HRT, menopause returns and will run its inevitable course. Any treatment only helps the symptoms.

So, what is menopause and why do we have to endure it?

Menopause is a natural decline in the body's reproductive hormones. The ovaries stop producing eggs, as the body eases out of its reproductive stage.

Menopause also represents the end of menstruation. Some women, especially those who've experienced premenstrual syndrome (PMS), embrace menopause for that reason alone. Others see it as exchanging one curse for another. Menstruation doesn't suddenly cease, it stops and starts, but gradually becomes less frequent. This stage is called *perimenopause* and can start around the age of forty. Perimenopause can last for a few years; the time frame is controlled by our genes. During the last stages of perimenopause, estrogen and progesterone decline rapidly and many women start to experience menopausal symptoms at that time.

When a woman has been twelve months without menstruation, she is considered menopausal.

Symptoms of menopause

- Mood swings

- Hot flashes

- Sweating

- Racing heart

- Headaches

- Muscle and joint pain

- Reduced sex drive

- Vaginal dryness

- Sleeping difficulties

Not all women will experience the whole range of symptoms; some will experience none, and others the full range. Menopausal symptoms may last for years and hot flashes are by far the most common symptom. There is a sensation of waves of extreme heat over the top half of the body.

Post menopause

Think the fun's over? Think again. Although the symptoms of menopause will eventually fade, due to a reduction in hormone levels, post-menopausal women have added health issues. However, these can be monitored and dealt with before they arise. Be on the lookout for:

- Decrease in bone density, with an increased risk of osteoporosis.

- Heart disease.

- Increased risk of Alzheimer's disease

- Poor skin elasticity and thinning hair.

- Weight gain

- Poor muscle strength and tone

I've addressed most of these in other chapters. Increased risk doesn't mean you *have* to suffer from any of the above.

Natural treatments for menopause

Here are some natural treatments specifically for hot flashes -

First avoid the things that trigger hot flashes. These can include:

- Spicy foods

- Stress

- Hot rooms

- Smoking

- Alcohol

- Coffee (don't shoot the messenger!)

Avoiding these triggers can go a long way to reducing hot flashes, however some may decide that doing without their morning coffee, or their favorite Thai curry, is not worth the sacrifice. I understand!

Hot flashes can also be minimized by standard menopause remedies –

Incorporate phytoestrogen foods into your diet. If you're already eating a clean diet, without processed foods or excess sugar, it's easy enough to add phytoestrogens to your diet. Phytoestrogens are plant-based estrogens that can have a similar effect to natural estrogen. There are pro and cons to increasing your estrogen levels during menopause. The advantages can be, reducing hot flashes, reducing the risk of some cancers, and lessening the risk of heart problems. On the other hand, women with a risk of breast cancer should completely avoid phytoestrogens. Some examples of phytoestrogens, include, soy products, Red Clover, Dong Quai, and Evening Primrose oil.

Omega-3 fats from fish or flaxseed, are indispensable for those experiencing menopausal symptoms. They protect the heart, prevent wrinkles, fight inflammation, prevent depression, and help keep bones strong. One daily capsule of Krill oil can ensure you get enough Omega-3.

Eat plenty of vegetables and a couple of pieces of fruit per day. These contain high amounts of dietary fiber, which will manage your appetite. They also contain antioxidants which slow the aging process and phytosterols that can balance hormones and lower cholesterol levels.

Herbal remedies

Black Cohosh –

Black cohosh was once thought to have an estrogenic effect on the body. However, recent research has disproved this. Many women have reported relief from menopausal symptoms from using this herb, so it's worth testing to see if it works for you. Black cohosh is similar in structure to *estradiol*, a hormone that occurs naturally in the human body. It contains a small amount of salicylic acid (used in aspirin), so can relieve pain and inflammation. The recommended dose is 20-40 mg tablets of the standardized extract, twice a day.

Red Clover -

Red clover is a phytoestrogen, so the warning for breast cancer patients apply. For everyone else, it's a safe herb that may alleviate menopausal symptoms, like hot flashes, sleeplessness, skin aging and thinning of the hair. Red clover acts quickly, but like most natural menopause remedies, it works well for some, but not for everyone. The recommended dose is 80 milligrams a day.

Dong Quai -

Dong Quai comes from traditional Chinese medicine. It has often been referred to as "female ginseng", due to its benefits on the symptoms of pre-menstrual tension, menopausal symptoms, and youthful appearance. Don Quai can also boost mood and is an excellent blood tonic. It is high in B vitamins and iron and can improve the appearance of skin and hair. Dong Quai is not safe for those who take blood thinning medication, or women with fibroids. As it's a phytoestrogen, women with breast cancer shouldn't take this herb.

Kava -

Kava used to be recommended for menopause symptoms, but research has shown it may cause liver cancer. It has been banned from sale in some countries, and I would not recommend it.

Evening Primrose Oil -

Evening Primrose oil (EPO) contains *gamma linoleic acid* (GLA) and has been used for hot flashes for many years. GLA can raise serotonin levels, benefitting mood, and helping skin retain moisture. It also can help with weight loss, by creating a feeling of fullness. Many studies have been done on EPO for hot flashes, and not all have been conclusive. However, many women have reported that EPO has reduced the severity of hot flashes considerably. For this reason, it is worth trying to see if it works for you. Evening primrose oil is available in capsules and should be kept refrigerated to keep the oil fresh. EPO should not be taken by anyone on blood-thinning or blood pressure medication. It can also react badly with some anti-depressant drugs, and should be discontinued for two weeks before a scheduled surgery. EPO may have an estrogenic in some women, so should be avoided by anyone with a high risk of breast cancer. In these cases, black currant seed oil – also a good source of GLA - may be substituted.

Wild Yam Cream -

Wild yam is a natural source of progesterone and can be substituted for synthetic progesterone cream. Consult your doctor first if progesterone cream has been medically prescribed. Wild yams contain a substance called *diosgenin*, a steroidal saponin. Wild Yam cream can be used together with estrogen to protect the uterus from the risk of endometrial cancer, that using estrogen alone can bring. *N.B - For those who've had a hysterectomy (removal of the uterus), progesterone isn't needed.*

Menopause can be a trying time, but natural remedies can ease the symptoms. Not all remedies work for all women, so trial and error will help find the right combination for you.

Sources:

http://www.webmd.com/menopause/guide/menopause-basics#1

https://www.betterhealth.vic.gov.au/health/conditionsandtreatments/menopause

http://www.healthline.com/health/menopause/menopause-facts#overview1

https://draxe.com/5-natural-remedies-menopause-relief/

https://draxe.com/red-clover/

https://www.drweil.com/health-wellness/health-centers/women/had-enough-wild-yams/

http://all-natural.com/womens-health/wildyam/

http://www.healthline.com/health/estradiol-test

http://www.healthline.com/health/dong-quai-ancient-mystery#overview1

http://www.34-menopause-symptoms.com/articles/dong-quai-does-it-work-for-treating-menopause.htm

http://www.livestrong.com/article/163621-benefits-of-evening-primrose-capsules/

https://www.betterhealth.vic.gov.au/health/conditionsandtreatments/menopause-and-complementary-therapies

Chapter 14 - Stress

"The time to relax is when you don't have time for it." – Sydney J. Harris

Stress is becoming natural in today's world, but when it takes over our lives, it becomes chronic. Chronic stress may be caused by excessive worry about events in our lives or those closest to us. Experiencing traumatic events may also lead to *post-traumatic stress disorder* (PTSD).

Chronic, or constant stress releases the stress hormones, cortisol, adrenaline, and noradrenaline. This can cause many unpleasant, and sometimes dangerous, symptoms:

- Elevated cholesterol

- High blood pressure

- Rapid heartbeat

- Inflamed circulatory system

- Compromised immunity

- Headache and migraine

- Higher blood glucose

- Muscle tension

- Increased abdominal fat

- Insomnia

- Skin problems. E.g. eczema and hives

- Impaired digestion

None of these looks like fun, and they're not! The effects of long-term chronic stress on the heart and blood vessels may lead eventually to a heart attack, especially after menopause. Our bodies contain less estrogen after menopause, putting us on the same level of risk as men of the same age. The liver produces more glucose under stress. This provides us with energy to fight or flee from whatever "emergency" our nervous system has identified. This may come in very handy when trying to escape from a dangerous dog but is not useful when the threat is in our minds. Then the body doesn't use up the extra glucose and it's re-absorbed, potentially causing problems for those whose glucose levels are already high. This can eventually lead to pre-diabetes, and after that, type 2 diabetes.

A weakened immune system opens the door to all kinds of disease. Stress hormones can slow the production of cytokines in the immune system, slowing its ability to fight infections, and even serious diseases.

Muscle tension increases under chronic stress, which can cause pain. The longer the stress drags on, the more likely the pain will become chronic. Realizing this can be a breakthrough to those suffering chronic pain, for which there seems to be no cause. In fact, here, the pain is acting as a warning signal.

"Studies have shown that chronic pain might not only be caused by physical injury but also by stress and emotional issues." - Dr. Susanne Babbel - Psychology Today.

How does muscle tension create chronic pain? If the muscles are contracted over a long period of time, they become tight and painful due to a lack of oxygen. Sometimes this can be completely unconscious when we're stressed. Please read the chronic pain chapter if this is a problem for you.

Stress can also affect our stomach and digestive system. Stress hormones slow the release of stomach acid, which means food may not be fully digested. Stress can also impact the intestines, so that they can't properly absorb nutrients from that food. If the stress continues, we may develop ulcers or disabling stomach pain.

Many of us older folk are working beyond retirement age; whether it's by necessity, or from choice. Work can add a lot of stress into our daily life, especially when it comes to lack of time. We try to get everything done by multitasking and rushing around in circles. Sometimes grandparents help their kids by babysitting, which can add extra pressure to their daily schedule. So, we really need a way to handle stress before it completely disrupts our lives. I've outlined the most effective 'stress busters' that I've found, and I'm hoping they'll help you too.

How to alleviate chronic stress

Breathe! It's amazing how simple breathing techniques can bring down stress, increase our energy and help us to sleep better. Deep breathing on its own, does help, but I've included a special breathing exercise below which is even more effective.

This breathing exercise, known as the *4-7-8 technique,* is an ancient meditation, thought to be used by yogis in India. It's extremely simple, but highly effective, and relaxes both the body and the mind. Simply find a comfortable position, inhale deeply through your nose for four seconds, hold for seven seconds, then exhale slowly through your mouth for eight seconds. Doing so expands the diaphragm, activating the *vagus* nerve. Not only does this practice calm you during a stressful day, but it's also a useful technique if you're having trouble sleeping. Using 4-7-8 breathing on a daily basis, trains the body to relax naturally, and the stress releasing benefits accumulate over time. If you have trouble doing this, reduce the timing and work up slowly. However always make sure the out-breath is longer than the in-breath.

Exercise - Bet you knew I'd slip this in here, didn't you? Regular exercise not only boosts mood and self-esteem, but it's also an excellent stress buster too. For dealing with stress, any type of exercise will work.

Sleep – Yes, I know it's hard to sleep when you're stressed; I've been there. There's nothing worse than staring at the ceiling while your mind whizzes around at a million miles an hour. If you're worried about anything, it always seems worse in those dark and lonely hours. Here are some quick tips on how to sleep better.

I'm assuming you know the standard advice that is always handed out regarding sleep, so I'll just mention them briefly here. Then I'll add a couple of "hacks" that I've used in the past.

Don't consume anything that contains caffeine after lunchtime. Caffeine can also be found in chocolate, sodas, energy drinks, cocoa, weight loss pills, and even decaffeinated coffee.

Make sure your bedroom is completely dark. This will ensure your melatonin levels remain high. For the same reason, don't watch TV or use any device with blue light for an hour before bed. The wavelengths from blue light are believed to suppress delta brainwaves and boost beta brainwaves, producing a state of alertness. Typical blue light appliances are backlit e-readers, laptops, and tablets. Reading a book or investing in blue light blocking glasses are better options.

Go to bed and wake up at the same time every morning, even on weekends. This establishes a sleep routine and resets your body clock. Try to perform the same tasks in the same order every night before bed. Both these actions will tell your sub-conscious mind that it's time for sleep.

Stop 'trying' to sleep. While this may sound absurd, by trying to sleep, you're actually telling yourself that you can't sleep, over and over again. The sub-conscious is extremely powerful, so tell yourself, "I am resting, and whether I sleep or not, doesn't matter."

Write your worries down before lying down to sleep. This gets them out of your head and onto a piece of paper. Then tell yourself, "I'll deal with them tomorrow". It's a simple way to tell your sub-conscious mind that there's no need to worry any more. Then, direct your thoughts onto something positive.

Listen to a podcast or similar media after switching off the light. This flies in the face of traditional advice but doing this has worked brilliantly for me. The reason being, your mind will focus the words and it will stop the endless mind chatter that keeps you awake, and stops you worrying about going to sleep. This works much better for me than listening to relaxation music.

Practice the 4-7-8 breathing exercise, as mentioned earlier in this chapter. It's magic for falling asleep, as well as getting back to sleep, if you tend to wake up during the night.

As Dr. Andrew Weil stated, *"It's the single best method that I've found for dealing with getting back to sleep if you wake up in the middle of the night,"*

Foods that can induce relaxation

There are certain foods, beverages and supplements that can help us relax. Here are the best ones:

Green Leafy Vegetables. Dark leafy greens are high in folate, which helps your body generate neurotransmitters, such as serotonin and dopamine. These neurotransmitters will improve your mood and trigger the relaxation response. Leafy greens also contain magnesium, a lack of which can induce anxiety and restlessness.

Magnesium can have a powerful calming effect on some people and is generally lacking in the typical diet. Start with 200 mg. a day, and work up to 400 mg. It's best taken at night, as it can have a sedating effect.

Green tea. Yes, it does have a small amount of caffeine, but this is more than offset by an amino acid called *theanine*. Theanine can relax the body without having a sedative effect. Theanine can increase the quality of sleep and prevent high blood pressure which tends to rise during stress.

Chamomile tea is known for its calming properties and is often included in natural sleep remedies.

Oatmeal and other healthy carbohydrates. Complex carbohydrate-rich foods raise serotonin levels, boosting your mood and helping you relax.

Eat foods which contain *tryptophan*. Tryptophan is an amino acid that is metabolized in the body to form serotonin. Foods containing tryptophan include turkey, chicken, milk, cheese, lentils, eggs, nuts, and seeds.

We can't totally avoid stress; it's part of the body's "fight or flight" response. Normal stress is fine and gives us the energy to deal with a temporary, stressful situation. Chronic stress is harmful but can be managed using the techniques mentioned above.

Sources:

https://www.psychologytoday.com/blog/somatic-psychology/201004/the-connections-between-emotional-stress-trauma-and-physical-pain

https://adaa.org/understanding-anxiety/related-illnesses/other-related-conditions/chronic-pain

http://www.apa.org/helpcenter/stress-body.aspx

https://www.mentalhelp.net/articles/the-long-term-consequences-of-negative-stress/

http://www.huffingtonpost.com/littlethingscom/the-incredible-way-your-e_b_7464472.html

https://my.clevelandclinic.org/health/articles/chronic-myofascial-pain-cmp

https://www.digitaltrends.com/mobile/does-blue-light-ruin-sleep-we-ask-an-expert/

http://articles.mercola.com/sites/articles/archive/2015/04/27/10-stress-relieving-superfoods.aspx

http://www.rd.com/health/healthy-eating/11-healthy-ways-to-destress-with-food/

https://www.mindbodygreen.com/0-17660/10-natural-tips-to-beat-chronic-stress.html

https://www.peoplespharmacy.com/2017/02/20/how-to-use-magnesium-to-get-to-sleep/

Bonus Chapter - Skin Care

"Beautiful young people are accidents of nature, but beautiful old people   are   works   of   art."
--Eleanor Roosevelt

I have never bought an expensive skin care product in my life. When I was young, it was because I couldn't afford to. Later it was because I knew I simply didn't have to.

I used to drool over those pretty jars of skin creams in the department stores, with their promises of eternal youth. I was twenty-five and stayed home to look after my daughter. My husband worked full time and took care of the mortgage, food, and electricity bills. There was always more month left than money.

I used to buy my skin care from health stores. They were quite basic back in those days. It was the early 1970s. I had a moisturizer for day use and a 'night' cream for before bed. I used *Dove* soap for cleansing.

Then I read in a woman's magazine, that sunscreen stopped the sun's ultraviolet rays from damaging skin and causing wrinkles, so I started using sunscreen. In those days, they were SPF-8 and oily. I had to apply it, wait ten minutes and blot off the excess oil before applying my make-up. It was tedious but I persevered.

I didn't realize it back then, but I was probably doing my skin a huge favor by *not* investing in expensive cosmetics. I'll explain why...

There are certain chemicals that almost all store-bought cosmetics contain. These serve several purposes.

- They preserve the life of the product

- They increase the viscosity (thickness) of lotions and creams

- They emulsify ingredients, which help oil and water combine

- They add foam to products such as cleansers and shampoos

- They strip oil from the skin to allow water to penetrate

If you're observant, you'll have noticed that the list of chemical functions above *has nothing to do with caring for your skin*. They are all about enhancing the product itself. But it gets worse. These chemicals can do a lot of harm, not only to your skin, but your internal organs too. They can affect hormonal balance and cause infertility. They have even been linked to cancer.

They're not just in cheap skin care products, but the most expensive ones too.

I once witnessed an interview between a talk show host and a representative of a large, well known cosmetics company. The host asked the representative the following question:

"... So, what are women actually paying for in your exclusive cosmetic range."

Momentarily flummoxed, the representative finally replied, "They are buying a dream."

Actually, they are buying a nightmare, but I digress...

There are many chemicals found in skin care. Many of them are harmless; many of them are not. So, the first part of this chapter will explain what not to use, and the second part is what to use instead. The following are the main ones to avoid.

Parabens

Parabens are cheap, and therefore, popular with cosmetic companies. They are used as a preservative; to increase the shelf-life of a product.

They preserve the appearance, fragrance, and ingredients. They are used across a wide range of products, face creams, cleansers and cosmetics.

The side effects of parabens are many. They include dryness, redness, burning and faster aging of the skin. Parabens can cause health problems as well. They have been linked to breast cancer, infertility in males, and increased estrogen in both sexes.

Because it is virtually impossible to avoid parabens completely, due to their presence in a huge range of products, it may be a good idea to read the label on your next skin care purchase and try to minimize your exposure.

Ethanolamines

You won't see this listed as such on any label. Here's what to look for. *DEA, TEA* and *MEA*. These are foaming agents and pH level controllers. They enable viscosity and allow a stable mix of oil and water. Ethanolamines are compounds of ammonia and are found mainly in body washes, shampoos, foaming cleansers, bubble baths and soaps.

Ethanolamines can lead to skin dryness, premature wrinkling, skin inflammation and irritation. Any product containing ethanolamines should be thoroughly rinsed off to minimize risk. Their risk increases with prolonged and continuous use.

Ethanolamines have also been linked to risk of cancer. Animal studies with DEA and MEA, in particular, have shown these chemicals to form tumors and to cause developmental abnormalities to an unborn fetus.

Sulphates

These are commonly called *Sodium Lauryl Sulfate, Ammonium Lauryl Sulfate, Sodium Laureth Sulfate or Ammonium Laureth Sulfate*.

Sulfates are an endocrine disrupting chemical which strips away the skin's protective barrier, allowing water to penetrate. This leaves your skin and hair vulnerable to surface damage and dehydration. Ultimately premature aging is accelerated, due to the damage caused by the loss of the skin's natural protective barrier.

These lovelies are mainly found in foaming cleansers and shampoos.

Have you ever washed your hair and found your scalp itchy afterward? You may think it's dandruff, but it's more likely to be sulphates attacking your skin. It's hard to find a store-bought shampoo without sulphates, as they produce all those lovely, scented bubbles! But shampoos without sulphates will cleanse your hair just as well. Sulfates can also cause hair loss, so try and find a sulfate-free shampoo. Check health stores and there are some nice ones on-line too.

Itchy scalps are bad enough, but when you wash your face, with a facewash which contains sulfates, it can dry your skin by stripping away the natural barrier. This can lead to premature wrinkling, crow's feet and burning of sensitive skin.

If you take one thing away from this chapter, it's this. Wash your face with a sulfate-free cleanser!

What else can sulfates do for us? They can cause weight gain and hormonal imbalances. They may even cause fertility problems.

There are other ingredients that are far less harmful, which can effectively cleanse the skin. These are - *sulfonate, disodium, cocamide, sodium cocosulfate or betaine.*

I'm sure a few of you may be thinking I'm being hysterical about this, and maybe you're right. Not everyone using these products will have a bad reaction. And no. You don't have to throw away those products already in your bathroom, just be aware when you replace them, and opt for safer ones.

We already live in a chemical filled world these days. They are everywhere. Why add to the load by using chemically based skincare?

Everything we put on out faces is absorbed by the skin's pores and can infiltrate our bloodstream.

You may be wondering why these chemical products are allowed to be sold. Although the screening process for medications is reasonably strict in most countries, the regulation of cosmetic and personal-care products is very lax in comparison. It's quite an easy process to have cosmetic products to be approved for commercial use. There are over one thousand ingredients that have been banned in cosmetic products in the European Union, at the time of writing. The number banned in the US is just ten!

In the end, it's a personal choice. I'm just making people aware that they *have* a choice.

A better choice for our skincare

You may be wondering where you can find skin-care products that are safe to use. There are two main options:

- Make your own

- Do some research and source chemical free products

I know we're all strapped for time, so making your own skin care might be low on your list of priorities. However, for those who are interested, home-made beauty products can be fun to make, cheap, and will be totally safe and irritant free. However, they won't contain preservatives, so will deteriorate with time. They will need to be refrigerated.

Ingredients for your home-made skin-products need not be expensive. In fact, you'll save a lot of money, especially if you've been using the expensive brands.

Some ingredients may already be in your fridge or kitchen cupboard. For instance, honey, coconut oil, oatmeal, and apple cider vinegar, avocado and lemons.

Others that may need to be bought are tea tree oil, aloe vera, jojoba oil, argon oil and shea butter. Olive oil is frequently used in natural products, but I have found personally, it isn't as effective as a moisturizer when compared to coconut oil.

Sourcing natural products can be time consuming, especially if you have to read the ingredients which are listed in small print. The easiest way is to do this on-line. There are several companies that make natural products these days.

Buying natural products will lessen your exposure to chemicals, but there are always a few in there. No store-bought product can be completely chemical free, or they would not last more than a few days on the shelf. However, it does mean that the manufacturer is more aware, and those chemicals that are in there, will probably be a lot less harmful.

Sources:

https://www.ncbi.nlm.nih.gov/pubmed/25128701

https://www.ncbi.nlm.nih.gov/pubmed/27581495

https://www.dermatocare.com/blog/Are-Parabens-in-cosmetic-contributing-to-Infertility-in-Males

https://www.ncbi.nlm.nih.gov/pubmed/17186576

Final Words

Committing to a healthy lifestyle isn't easy. It involves making some sacrifices; giving up things that you may think you can't live without. I'm here to tell you that you can. Do I follow this advice all the time without fail? No. I'm human. I will occasionally splurge on a chocolate bar, or something else sweet. It's what we do 95% of the time that counts.

I hope you found this book empowering. I certainly found that writing it empowered me. It was a lot of work and research, but I discovered new things, because the health landscape is always changing. It reminded me of things I already knew but had let slide. Inconvenient truths!

Health is a choice. Make it yours.

Wishing you a long and healthy life!

With love,

Wendy Owen

If you have enjoyed this book, I'd be delighted if you could go to Amazon and leave me a review. Here's the link - https://www.amazon.com/dp/B073QHCKRJ/

Thank you!

Made in the USA
Coppell, TX
07 January 2022